T0202894

SBAs for the FRCR 2A

SBAs for the FRCR 2A

Edited by

Stuart Currie

Emma Rowbotham

Shishir Karthik

Christopher Wilkinson

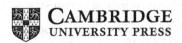

CAMBRIDGE
UNIVERSITY PRESS

University Printing House, Cambridge CB2 8BS, United Kingdom

One Liberty Plaza, 20th Floor, New York, NY 10006, USA

477 Williamstown Road, Port Melbourne, VIC 3207, Australia

314-321, 3rd Floor, Plot 3, Splendor Forum, Jasola District Centre, New Delhi - 110025, India

103 Penang Road, #05-06/07, Visioncrest Commercial, Singapore 238467

Cambridge University Press is part of the University of Cambridge.

It furthers the University's mission by disseminating knowledge in the pursuit of
education, learning and research at the highest international levels of excellence.

www.cambridge.org
Information on this title: www.cambridge.org/9780521156448

First published 2010

A catalogue record for this publication is available from the British Library

Library of Congress Cataloging in Publication data
SBAs for the FRCR 2A / edited by Stuart Currie ... [et al.].
     p. ; cm.
  Includes bibliographical references and index.
  ISBN 978-0-521-15644-8 (pbk.)
  1. Radiography, Medical–Problems, exercises, etc.   2. Radiography, Medical–
Licenses–Great Britain–Examinations–Study guides.   I. Currie, Stuart, Dr.
  [DNLM: 1. Radiography–Examination Questions. WN 18.2 S276 2010]
  RC78.15.S33 2010
  616.07´572076–dc22

                                                                    2009044697

ISBN 978-0-521-15644-8 Paperback

Additional resources for this publication at www.cambridge.org/9780521156448

....

Every effort has been made in preparing this book to provide accurate and
up-to-date information which is in accord with accepted standards and practice
at the time of publication. Although case histories are drawn from actual cases,
every effort has been made to disguise the identities of the individuals involved.
Nevertheless, the authors, editors and publishers can make no warranties that the
information contained herein is totally free from error, not least because clinical
standards are constantly changing through research and regulation. The authors,
editors and publishers therefore disclaim all liability for direct or consequential
damages resulting from the use of material contained in this book. Readers
are strongly advised to pay careful attention to information provided by the
manufacturer of any drugs or equipment that they plan to use.

To our loving families

Contents

Contributors

Dr Dominic Barron
Consultant Radiologist, Leeds Teaching Hospitals NHS Trust, Leeds, UK.

Dr Stuart Currie
Department of Radiology, Leeds General Infirmary, Leeds, UK.

Dr Shishir Karthik
Department of Radiology, Leeds General Infirmary, Leeds, UK.

Dr Emma Rowbotham
Department of Radiology, Leeds General Infirmary, Leeds, UK.

Dr Damian Tolan
Consultant Radiologist, Leeds Teaching Hospitals NHS Trust, Leeds, UK.

Dr Christopher Wilkinson
Department of Radiology, Leeds General Infirmary, Leeds, UK.

Preface

For many, single best answer (SBA) questions represent a novel mode of testing, and with new concepts often come concern and anxiety. The best way to alleviate these feelings is through familiarisation and preparation.

Working through large textbooks can be laborious and time-consuming, and can often leave one feeling that they have achieved very little. What's needed is a book that provides the FRCR candidate with a breadth of knowledge through a myriad of examination practice questions that are supported with concise yet accurate answers.

This is where this book excels!

With 360 'life-like' examination questions which cover the key concepts of each of the six Part 2A modules, this book is a must for all FRCR candidates. New modalities and their increasing role in the management of patients are addressed. What's more, because each question encompasses a new radiological scenario and is accompanied by reasoned answers, the reader is quickly left with a sense of achievement during their exam revision.

This book is perfect for 'sneaking' revision into busy working lives and for those candidates who demand more, the references that accompany the answers permit further knowledge acquisition.

An abundance of practice questions and detailed answers with references! This book is an essential FRCR revision companion.

Introduction

Congratulations on passing the FRCR Part 1!

Now for Part 2A: six modules of single best answer (SBA) questions. Don't panic! Remember lots of candidates pass every year, so success is achievable.

We found the best way to pass was to practise, practise and practise mock questions. Unfortunately, many books pose irrelevant questions, or offer little in the way of answers or explanation. This contradicts the purpose of a revision book, which is meant to help avoid the laborious task of sifting through countless textbook pages.

With these failings in mind, we have written a book which covers the relevant information of all six modules and provides concise yet informative referenced answers.

Go on, test yourself! Start now and never look back. Success is just around the corner. Good luck!

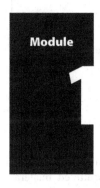

Module 1

Cardiothoracic and vascular – Questions

1. A 50 year old male presents with a history of occasional haemoptysis and exertional shortness of breath which has been getting progressively worse. Plain chest radiograph demonstrates bibasal reticular shadowing with volume loss. HRCT demonstrates bibasal fibrosis and traction bronchiectasis. Incidental note is made of a patulous oesophagus. Which of the following is the most likely cause?
   a. Tuberculosis
   b. SLE
   c. Rheumatoid arthritis
   d. Wegener's granulomatosis
   e. Scleroderma

2. A 35 year old woman presents with chest infection and pyrexia and the plain film reveals dense lobar consolidation with bulging fissures. The likely micro-organism is:
   a. *Legionella pneumophila*
   b. *Pneumocystis carinii*
   c. *Staphylococcus*
   d. *Streptococcus*
   e. *Klebsiella*

3. A 40 year old has a routine chest radiograph as a part of pre-immigration work up. This demonstrates a mass on the left with loss of the upper left heart border. The descending aorta can, however, be seen despite the mass. Which of the following is the most likely location of the mass?
   a. Apico-posterior segment
   b. Lingula
   c. Anterior segment of the upper lobe
   d. Posterior basal segment of the lower lobe
   e. Lateral basal segment of the lower lobe

4. In an investigation for lung malignancy, all of the following may produce a false positive result on a PET-CT except:
   a. Pulmonary hamartoma
   b. Intralobar sequestration
   c. Tuberculosis
   d. Pneumonia
   e. Scarring

5. A 70 year old man, previously working in a ship-building yard, presents with progressive breathlessness. Chest radiograph demonstrates bilateral calcified pleural plaque disease

with volume loss. Lung function shows a restrictive pattern. HRCT reveals pulmonary fibrosis. The most likely site of these changes would be:

a. Perihilar
b. Apical
c. Peribronchial
d. Subpleural
e. Fissural

6. A 35 year old man undergoes autologous bone marrow transplantation following successful treatment of lymphoma. Two weeks later he develops scattered bilateral progressive breathlessness and dry cough. HRCT demonstrates several areas of bilateral ground glass changes with associated reticular changes, but no effusions. What is the most likely explanation?

a. Angioinvasive aspergillosis
b. Lymphoid interstitial pneumonia
c. CMV pneumonia
d. Drug toxicity
e. Pulmonary oedema

7. A 67 year old man presents with abdominal discomfort three months after endovascular repair of an abdominal aortic aneurysm. The patient undergoes a non-contrast CT followed by an arterial phase study. There is high attenuation on the non-contrast study between the stent and the aortic wall, which enhances further in the arterial phase. The graft itself is intact, as are the attachment sites. Which of the following is the most likely cause for the appearance?

a. Type I endoleak
b. Type II endoleak
c. Type III endoleak
d. Graft infection
e. Dissection

8. A 16 year old with headache and hypertension has a chest radiograph which demonstrates plain radiographic signs of coarctation of the aorta. Further investigations reveal anomalous post-coarctation origin of the right subclavian artery. The ribs most likely to demonstrate inferior rib notching would be:

a. Left third to ninth ribs
b. Bilateral third to ninth ribs
c. Right third to ninth ribs
d. Bilateral first and second ribs
e. Left first and second ribs

9. A 38 year old man with progressive dyspnoea and chest pain undergoes an echocardiogram which reveals a pedunculated intracardiac mass which is hypointense to myocardium on T1-weighted images and markedly hyperintense on T2-weighted images. The most likely intracardiac location of the lesion would be:

a. Right atrium
b. Right ventricle
c. Left atrium
d. Under-surface of tricuspid valve
e. Anterior papillary muscle

2

10. A 56 year old female is found to have a small, well-defined anterior mediastinal mass on a chest radiograph which demonstrates homogeneous soft-tissue density with some peripheral calcification on CT. On MRI it is isointense to skeletal muscle on T1-weighted images and slightly increased signal on T2-weighted images. It is most likely to be:
    a. Thymic cyst
    b. Thymoma
    c. Thymolipoma
    d. Thymic hyperplasia
    e. Thymic carcinoma

11. A 51 year old man with long standing history of an erosive arthropathy of the acromio-clavicular joints and bilateral arthropathy in his hands subsequently develops progressive shortness of breath. The most likely abnormality on his chest radiograph would be:
    a. Cavitating nodules
    b. Peripheral basal reticulonodular shadowing
    c. Cardiomegaly
    d. Bronchiectasis
    e. Pleural effusion

12. A 22 year old is diagnosed with tuberculosis. Which of the following features will make a diagnosis of primary tuberculosis more likely?
    a. Mediastinal enlargement
    b. Septal thickening
    c. Upper zone cavitation
    d. Miliary nodules
    e. Apical consolidation

13. A 26 year old man suffers a blunt injury to his chest in a road traffic accident. The most common abnormality seen on CT as a result of blunt thoracic injury is:
    a. Pneumothorax
    b. Pulmonary laceration
    c. Haemothorax
    d. Tracheo-bronchial injuries
    e. Pulmonary contusion

14. A 26 year old undergoes a routine chest radiograph as part of the Australian residency application. The left upper lobe is hyperlucent and hyperexpanded and a lobular mass is demonstrated adjacent to the left hilum. CT reveals the presence of a dilated bronchus containing a plug of soft tissue. The surrounding lung is emphysematous. The most likely diagnosis is:
    a. Central carcinoid tumour
    b. Bronchogenic cyst
    c. Bronchial atresia
    d. Cystic adenomatoid malformation
    e. Congenital lobar emphysema

15. A 58 year old man with pancreatic cancer presents with recurrent pulmonary emboli despite adequate anticoagulation. He is shown on this admission to also have a right femoral DVT. He subsequently undergoes an IVC filter placement. Following a flush

injection in the IVC, injecting contrast at which of the following site is essential prior to stent placement?

a. Right hepatic vein
b. Left renal vein
c. Right common iliac vein
d. Right renal vein
e. Left common iliac vein

16. A 40 year old man presents with worsening breathlessness, fever and chills following a visit to an aviary earlier in the day. HRCT is most likely to demonstrate:

a. Mid-zone interstitial lines
b. Areas of air-space shadowing
c. Pleural effusions
d. Lymphadenopathy
e. Crazy paving

17. The staging chest CT of a 40 year old man with a known primary malignancy demonstrates cavitating pulmonary metastases. The least likely type of primary lesion would be:

a. Squamous cell carcinoma
b. Malignant melanoma
c. Renal cell cancer
d. Sarcomas
e. Colonic carcinoma

18. A 25 year old woman with a longstanding history of non-erosive arthritis of the hands and a malar rash presents with progressive breathlessness and respiratory dysfunction. Blood serology demonstrates anti-DNA antibodies. Which of the following is the most common feature on the chest radiograph?

a. Pleural effusion
b. Consolidation
c. Cavitating nodules
d. Pulmonary oedema
e. Pulmonary fibrosis

19. A 40 year old man with a known malignancy presents with pericardial metastases and pericardial effusion. The metastatic deposits are high signal on T1-weighted imaging. Which is the likely primary diagnosis?

a. Lymphoma
b. Lung cancer
c. Melanoma
d. Fibrosarcoma
e. Colorectal cancer

20. The diagnostic role of CT in patients with pulmonary emboli is well established, but a prognostic role is being proposed as well. Which of the following has the most widely accepted prognostic value?

a. PA clot burden score
b. Leftward bowing of the intraventricular septum
c. Reflux of contrast into the IVC
d. RV/LV diameter ratio
e. PA diameter measurement

21. A 55 year old man has a repeat chest radiograph which demonstrates a persistent patch of consolidation four months after a previous radiograph. Bronchioloalveolar carcinoma (BAC) is suspected. Which of the following makes the diagnosis less likely?
   a. Low attenuation consolidation
   b. Negative PET-CT
   c. Central location
   d. Long history of smoking
   e. Associated cavitation

22. A 62 year old man presents with right shoulder pain which radiates down his arm. A plain radiograph confirms the presence of a right apical mass with destruction of the surrounding ribs. CT-guided biopsy is performed and is likely to reveal:
   a. Large cell lung cancer
   b. Squamous cell cancer
   c. Small cell lung cancer
   d. Adenocarcinoma
   e. Carcinoid

23. A 25 year old man has a routine chest radiograph prior to a work permit application. It demonstrates a well-defined, rounded mediastinal mass. Which of the following features on CT would make a diagnosis of bronchogenic cyst less likely?
   a. Soft-tissue density
   b. Thick wall
   c. Precarinal location
   d. Communication with tracheal lumen
   e. Unilocularity

24. A 45 year old man presents with a history of cough and occasional haemoptysis. Plain chest radiograph demonstrates a right paracardiac shadow with loss of the right heart border. Bronchoscopy demonstrates an endoluminal obstructive mass. The most likely site of the lesion would be:
   a. Right upper lobe anterior segmental bronchus
   b. Right lower lobe lateral basal segmental bronchus
   c. Bronchus intermedius
   d. Right upper lobe posterior segmental bronchus
   e. Right middle lobe bronchus

25. A 54 year old man presents with breathlessness and palpitations. Clinical examination reveals a mid-diastolic murmur with presystolic accentuation. Echocardiography confirms the presence of a mobile intracardiac mass in the left atrium attached to the septum by means of a stalk. Which of the following is the most likely feature of the lesion on MRI?
   a. Hypointense relative to myocardium on T1-weighted images
   b. Uniform hyperintense to myocardium on T2-weighted images
   c. Uniform enhancement following gadolinium
   d. Hyperintense to blood pool and hypointense to myocardium on steady-state free precession (SSFP) images
   e. Prolapse of the mass through the mitral valve, best demonstrated on the short axis views

26. A 34 year old IV drug abuser presents with fever, rigors and back pain. Blood cultures reveal staphylococcal septicaemia. CT demonstrates a mycotic aneurysm. Which of the following is the most likely CT feature?
    a. Fusiform shape
    b. Perianeurysmal soft-tissue mass
    c. Pseudoaneurysm
    d. Periaortic gas collection
    e. Mural thrombus

27. An area of abnormality is noted within the juxtahepatic IVC of a patient with cirrhosis undergoing an MR scan. The area is hyperintense on T1-weighted imaging, and appears as a filling defect on three-dimensional fat-suppressed volume-interpolated breathhold sequence. Appearances vary in shape and location on different images. The abnormality is likely to represent:
    a. Flowing blood
    b. Thrombus
    c. Tumour thrombus
    d. Artefact due to aortic pulsation
    e. Pseudolipoma

28. A 60 year old female underwent a right pneumonectomy for bronchogenic carcinoma. Which feature on plain chest radiograph would be a cause of worry seven days after surgery?
    a. A sequential increase in the fluid level
    b. Shift of the previously central trachea to the right
    c. Shift of the previously central trachea to the left
    d. Elevation of the right hemi-diaphragm
    e. Shift of the cardiac silhouette to the right

29. A 22 year old asthmatic presents with recurrent wheeze and productive cough with expectoration of brown sputum. Plain chest radiograph demonstrates multiple pulmonary infiltrates. Which of the following appearances on HRCT would be the most appropriate for acute allergic bronchopulmonary aspergillosis?
    a. Finger-in-glove opacity
    b. Thick-walled cavity
    c. Pleural thickening with or without an effusion
    d. Endobronchial mass with distal atelectasis
    e. Tree-in-bud appearance

30. A 36 year old female with history of pelvic pain and severe dysmenorrhoea undergoes a pelvic ultrasound examination which reveals uterine fibroid disease. Which of the following imaging features would be associated with the best outcome following uterine artery embolisation?
    a. Submucosal location
    b. Subserosal location
    c. Associated adenomyosis
    d. Calcification
    e. Multiple fibroids

31. A young man presents with progressive productive cough and halitosis. He had severe pneumonia as a child. Plain chest radiograph demonstrates bronchial dilatation and

bronchial wall thickening with some volume loss. Which of the following HRCT findings is the most sensitive finding for bronchiectasis?
a. Air trapping
b. Mucous-filled dilated bronchi
c. Bronchial wall thickening
d. Bronchi seen in the subpleural region
e. Lack of bronchial tapering

32. A 35 year old female presents with generalised malaise and cough, occasionally bringing up grape-skin-like material. Blood screen reveals eosinophilia. The patient has a history of travel to several countries worldwide. Which of the following plain film features is unlikely?
a. Homogenous ovoid opacity
b. Cyst with a fluid level
c. Bilateral opacities
d. Calcification
e. Lower zone location

33. A 33 year old male patient suffering from AIDS presents with constitutional symptoms and dry cough. His CD4 count is 150. HRCT is least likely to show:
a. Pleural effusion
b. Ground glass changes
c. Bilateral interstitial infiltrates
d. Diffuse alveolar infiltrates
e. Pneumatocoeles

34. A 26 year old female patient with an optic nerve tumour and café-au-lait spots presents with exertional breathlessness. Imaging of the chest is most likely to reveal which of the following?
a. Multiple small lower lobe cysts
b. Emphysema
c. Lower zone fibrosis
d. Thick-walled cavities in the upper zone
e. Asymmetrical upper zone fibrosis

35. A 52 year old with cardiomyopathy is referred for delayed contrast-enhanced cardio-vascular MR (DE-CMR). The following are all false except:
a. An inversion recovery pulse of an appropriate TI is applied to nullify the signal from the ischaemic myocardium
b. A long TI would nullify the signal from both the normal and diseased tissue
c. A TI of 200 ms would nullify the signal intensity from the normal myocardium
d. Imaging should be commenced immediately after contrast injection
e. The images are T1-weighted ECG-gated fast spin-echo sequences with an inversion recovery sequence

36. In the same patient (with cardiomyopathy), which underlying cause and corresponding enhancement pattern are inappropriate?
a. Ischaemic cardiomyopathy – subendocardial pattern in a coronary artery territory
b. Early myocarditis – patchy, focal subendocardial pattern

c. Hypertrophic cardiomyopathy – patchy multifocal changes, commonly the right ventricular free wall and its junction with the interventricular septum

d. Amyloidosis – global and diffuse, commonly subendocardial

e. Dilated cardiomyopathy – midwall myocardial enhancement

37. A 30 year old man has a routine chest radiograph which reveals a small soft-tissue shadow resulting in loss of part of the mid-descending aortic outline. Which of the following is the most likely cause?

a. Thymoma in the left lobe of thymus

b. Hilar lymphadenopathy

c. Lingular collapse

d. Intercostal schwannoma

e. Teratoma

38. A 68 year old miner develops an irregular opacity in the upper zone on plain chest radiograph. Which imaging feature would be more in favour of malignancy than progressive massive fibrosis (PMF)?

a. Peripheral enhancement on contrast-enhanced MR

b. Peripheral location on axial images

c. Presence of calcification

d. High signal on T2-weighted images

e. Avid lesion on PET-CT

39. A 36 year old asthmatic attends an outpatient respiratory clinic complaining of recent increasing dyspnoea. Bloods show an elevated white cell count and eosinophilia. Chest radiograph reveals multiple areas of ill-defined peripherally based consolidation. Subsequent chest radiographs over the coming week show the consolidation to resolve in places but commence in other previously unaffected areas. The most likely cause is:

a. Alveolar sarcoidosis

b. Bronchioalveolar carcinoma

c. Acute eosinophilic pneumonia

d. Chronic eosinophilic pneumonia

e. Loffler syndrome

40. The plain chest radiograph of a 52 year old male presenting with cough and haemoptysis reveals a veil-like opacity over the left upper zone. CT reveals an endobronchial lesion in the left upper lobe bronchus causing lobar collapse. Bronchoscopic biopsy is least likely to reveal:

a. Squamous cell carcinoma

b. Carcinoid

c. Lymphoma

d. Metastatic renal cell cancer

e. Bronchioloalveolar carcinoma

41. A 60 year old man who recently suffered a haemorrhagic stroke develops pulmonary emboli. He is referred for an IVC filter insertion and angiography is performed prior to this. The usual reasons for doing so would be all of the following except:

a. To identify the renal veins

b. To identify the hepatic veins

    c. To size the IVC

    d. To rule out the presence of a left IVC

    e. To evaluate for the presence of an IVC thrombus

42. A 22 year old female patient with a known phakomatosis presents with anaemia and hypotension. CT angiogram reveals evidence of active bleeding in some of the multiple areas of low attenuation (approximately –20) seen scattered throughout both her kidneys. Which of the following features may be seen on chest CT?

    a. Multiple pulmonary AVMs

    b. Multiple bilateral small cysts

    c. Mediastinal mass

    d. Thin-walled upper zone bullae

    e. Cardiac rhabdomyomas

43. A 33 year old female patient presents with a longstanding history of fever, dry cough and weight loss. The chest radiograph reveals mediastinal lymphadenopathy. Blood investigations reveal hypercalcemia and elevated angiotensin-converting enzyme (ACE). Which of the following appearances of lymphadenopathy on CT would be the least likely feature in favour of the clinical diagnosis?

    a. Bilateral hilar lymphadenopathy

    b. Egg-shell calcification

    c. Predominant involvement of the right paratracheal lymph nodes

    d. Lymphadenopathy without any parenchymal involvement

    e. Posterior mediastinal lymph nodes

44. The HRCT of a 35 year old patient with shortness of breath and reticulonodular disease pattern on plain chest radiograph reveals cavitating nodules with interstitial septal thickening. Which of the following diagnoses is the least likely?

    a. Lymphangioleiomyomatosis

    b. Langerhans' cell histiocytosis

    c. Wegener's granulomatosis

    d. Sarcoidosis

    e. Rheumatoid lung

45. Eight days after lung transplantation for alpha-1 antitrypsin deficiency, a 45 year old man develops pyrexia, breathlessness and desaturation. HRCT reveals perihilar hetero-genous opacities and ground glass changes with new pleural effusion and septal thickening. Which of the following is the most likely cause?

    a. Reperfusion oedema

    b. Acute rejection

    c. Anastomotic dehiscence

    d. Post-transplantation PCP infection

    e. Hyperacute rejection

46. A 45 year old female patient with history of rheumatic fever as a child presents with progressive shortness of breath and paroxysmal nocturnal dyspnoea. Clinical examin-ation reveals a pansystolic murmur associated with a mid-diastolic murmur with presystolic accentuation best heard over the cardiac apex. Clinical examination and

plain film do not reveal evidence of heart failure, but several features of left atrial enlargement are noted. Which of the following is not one of those?

a. Double atrial shadow on the right
b. Straightening of the right heart border
c. Elevation of the left main bronchus
d. Splaying of the carina
e. Displacement of the descending aorta to the left

47. A 70 year old man undergoes surgery for AAA. Two weeks following surgery, he is readmitted to the A&E department with abdominal pain and fever. Palpation of the abdomen suggests a pulsatile mass. A CT angiogram is performed, which does not demonstrate contrast extravasation. Which of the features on CT angiogram would be most worrisome?

a. Presence of a pseudoaneurysm
b. Periaortic soft tissue
c. Thickening of a fluid-filled third part of the duodenum
d. Some ectopic gas in the vicinity
e. Loss of fat plane between the grafted aorta and the adjacent duodenum

48. A seven year old boy with no known medical history presents with hypertension and postprandial abdominal pain. CT reveals an abnormality in the abdominal vasculature. Subsequent angiogram demonstrates occlusion of the coeliac axis and superior mesenteric artery and tapering of the mid-aorta. Delayed imaging shows vessel reconstitution through collaterals. The most likely diagnosis is?

a. Takayasu arteritis
b. Midaortic syndrome
c. Neurofibromatosis
d. Marfan's syndrome
e. Syphilitic aortitis

49. A patient with a known collagen vascular disease has pulmonary fibrosis. HRCT reveals bilateral lower lobe bronchiectasis. Which collagen vascular disease is most likely?

a. Sjogren syndrome
b. Progressive systemic sclerosis
c. SLE
d. Rheumatoid arthritis
e. Dermatomyositis

50. A 30 year old female patient with a history of recurrent lower respiratory tract infections as a child presents with cough and dyspnoea. Chest radiograph demonstrates a smaller hyperlucent left lung. Which of the following features is unlikely to be seen on HRCT?

a. Air trapping
b. Small left hemithorax
c. Diminished size of pulmonary vessels
d. Bronchiectasis
e. Left hilar enlargement

51. A 60 year old man presents with a 6 month history of shortness of breath, wheeze and a recent episode of haemoptysis. Plain chest radiograph reveals partial right middle and

lower lobe collapse. This is further confirmed on CT which also suggests an endo-bronchial lesion in the bronchus intermedius. It is FDG-avid on PET-CT scan. Bronchoscopy reveals a smooth submucosal lesion. The histopathology of the lesion is most likely to be:

a. Mucoepidermoid carcinoma
b. Atypical carcinoid
c. Renal cell carcinoma metastasis
d. Adenoid cystic carcinoma
e. Squamous cell papilloma

52. A 36 year old female awaiting liver transplantation undergoes routine pre-operative planning ultrasound examination of the abdomen. Whilst the rest of the abdomen is normal, a 4 cm splenic artery aneurysm is seen, which is subsequently confirmed on CT. Which of the following would be the preferred course of action?

a. Follow-up ultrasound scan in a year's time
b. Referral to the surgeons for a splenectomy
c. Thrombin injection of the aneurysm
d. Endoscopic ligation of the aneurysm
e. Coil embolisation of the aneurysm

53. A 59 year old male presents with left shoulder pain and tingling in his fingers. Plain chest radiograph reveals the presence of a left apical mass with some rib destruction. CT confirms the presence of a superior sulcus tumour at the left apex with no evidence of nodal or distant metastasis. The patient is referred for a MR scan to assess resect-ability. Which of the following is appropriate?

a. Coronal T1-weighted images are best to identify involvement of the brachial plexus
b. T2-weighted images are vital to assess resectability and should be performed first
c. Axial images are best to assess spinal canal and foraminal involvement
d. Use of intravenous contrast is necessary to identify the subclavian vessels and their relation to the brachial plexus and the tumour
e. Imaging is usually performed using a body coil

54. A 60 year old hypertensive man presents with sudden-onset severe inter-scapular pain. CT reveals a high attenuation crescent in the wall of the proximal ascending aorta with inward displacement of part of the calcific wall, which extends just up to the brachio-cephalic artery. Post-contrast scan does not demonstrate leak of contrast into the crescentic area or mediastinum. The patient is haemodynamically stable. The next appropriate course of action is:

a. Urgent cardiothoracic referral
b. Contact the interventional radiologist for consideration of endovascular stenting
c. Follow-up scan after 24 hours
d. Medical treatment aimed at controlling blood pressure
e. Emergency cardiac MRI

55. A 30 year old female with uncontrolled hypertension undergoes an MR angiogram of the renal arteries. This reveals bilateral renal artery abnormalities. The most likely abnormality is:

a. Bilateral ostial stenosis
b. Bilateral long segment stenosis

   c. Intrarenal aneurysms

   d. Atretic renal arteries with extensive collateralisation

   e. Multiple stenoses of the mid portion of the renal arteries

56. A 45 year old woman with severe portal hypertension and variceal bleeding is referred for a trans-jugular intrahepatic porto-systemic shunt (TIPSS) procedure following the failure of endoscopic procedures in controlling the bleeding. Which of the following is the most appropriate regarding TIPSS?

   a. The middle hepatic vein is the preferred route of access to the portal vein

   b. The right portal vein is usually posterior to the right hepatic vein

   c. Flow of contrast towards the porta hepatis usually indicates puncture of the biliary tree

   d. The gradient across the shunt should be less than 20 mmHg

   e. Stenosis tends to occur in the portal vein

57. Following a deceleration injury in a road traffic accident, a young man presents to the A&E department with shock, chest wall contusion and severe chest pain. An aortic injury is suspected. Which of the following is least likely?

   a. A normal chest radiograph has high negative predictive value

   b. Aortic injury is the usual cause of mediastinal haematoma

   c. The aorta just beyond the left subclavian artery is the most common site of injury

   d. Aortic rupture is usually circumferential

   e. A non-contrast CT scan has a high negative predictive value in the absence of demonstrable mediastinal haematoma

58. A 45 year old man with a known atrial septal defect (ASD) presents with breathlessness and mild cyanosis. Clinical examination reveals a loud second heart sound and a prominent parasternal heave, but no signs of heart failure. Echocardiogram demonstrates a shunt reversal. Which of the following is not a usual feature on the imaging?

   a. Paucity of peripheral pulmonary vasculature

   b. Enlarged central PA

   c. Right ventricular hypertrophy

   d. Dilated pulmonary veins

   e. Linear calcification of the main pulmonary arteries

59. A 60 year old man presents with progressive breathlessness. The plain chest radiograph reveals reticular shadowing in the right lower zone, but is otherwise unremarkable. HRCT demonstrates the presence of beaded thickening of the interlobular septae forming a polygonal reticular network in the right lower lobe with central dots within. There is also a small pleural effusion. Which of the following is the most likely cause?

   a. Sarcoidosis

   b. Bronchogenic carcinoma

   c. Heart failure

   d. Extrinsic allergic alveolitis

   e. Fibrosing alveolitis

60. A 32 year old patient with congenital heart disease is referred for a cardiac MR examination. Regarding cardiac MR imaging, which of the following applies?

a. Dark rim artefacts are typically seen on the epicardial aspect on perfusion imaging
b. Radiofrequency artefacts are typically sporadic and transient, affecting few images in a series
c. Field inhomogeneity artefacts are more common on a 3T scanner than a 1.5T scanner
d. Of the two cine MR imaging techniques, at the same bandwidth, image acquisition is quicker with an SSFP sequence than spoiled GRE imaging
e. Prospective gating is preferred for assessing diastolic dysfunction

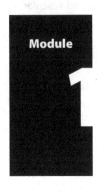

Cardiothoracic and vascular – Answers

1. e. Scleroderma
Whilst haemoptysis may be a presentation in tuberculosis and Wegener's and bibasal fibrosis maybe seen in all of the above except tuberculosis (where apical fibrosis is the more likely feature), scleroderma is the only condition resulting in a patulous lower oesophageal sphincter, oesophageal shortening and stricture formation.
(Ref: Dahnert p. 863)

2. e. Klebsiella
Klebsiella causes a dense pneumonia with bulging of fissures often associated with an empyema. Pneumococcal pneumonitis can also mimic this.
(Ref: Dahnert p. 504)

3. b. Lingula
This is an example of the silhouette sign where an anteriorly located lingular mass results in loss of the upper left heart border but preservation of the outline of the posterior descending aorta.
(Ref: Grainger & Allison p. 319)

4. b. Intralobar sequestration
Active tuberculosis, consolidation, atypical pulmonary hamartomas and scars may cause false positive results. Uncomplicated sequestration will not demonstrate FDG uptake.
(Ref: Park CM *et al.* Tumors in the tracheobronchial tree: CT and FDG PET features. *Radiographics* 2009; 29: 55–71)

5. d. Subpleural
Pulmonary fibrosis associated with asbestos exposure is seen mainly in a subpleural distribution towards the lung bases.
(Ref: Dahnert p. 464)

6. d. Drug toxicity
Post transplant pulmonary complications may develop in up to 40–60% of patients. In the first two weeks or so after transplantation, neutropaenia is the underlying cause for most of these. Angioinvasive aspergillosis presents in the first two to three weeks, usually as multiple ground glass nodules with or without cavitation and peribronchiolar consolidation.

Lymphoid interstitial pneumonia (LIP) is a late-phase complication usually seen more than three months after transplantation and may be an indication of chronic graft-versus-host response. CMV pneumonia may manifest at any time in the first 100 days after transplantation.

Multiple nodules with associated ground glass changes or consolidation are usually seen, but reticular change is not a feature. Pulmonary oedema is also seen in the neutropaenic phase in the first two to three weeks. Whilst ground glass changes and interstitial lines are seen in pulmonary oedema, associated pleural effusion is common.

Drug toxicity due to a variety of chemotherapeutic agents is seen in the neutropaenic phase as a combination of ground glass and reticular changes.
(Ref: Dahnert p. 469)

7. b. Type II endoleak
Type II endoleaks are due to retrograde flow from the small branches of the aorta such as the lumbar arteries. A Type I endoleak is due to a seal failure at either end, type III is due to a defect in the graft and type IV is due to graft porosity.
(Ref: Dahnert p. 618)

8. a. Left third to ninth ribs
Due to the anomalous origin of the right subclavian artery from the post-coarctation segment, there is no collateral flow to the intercostal arteries on the right. Subsequently, there is no right-sided rib notching.
(Ref: Dahnert p. 630)

9. c. Left atrium
The case describes an atrial myxoma, which is more common in the left atrium (75–80% of cases). These tumours are usually attached to the inter-atrium septum.
(Ref: Dahnert p. 646)

10. b. Thymoma
This case describes the typical features of a thymoma. Thymic hyperplasia and thymic carcinoma are usually ill-defined abnormalities. The signal from the lesion is not typical for a thymic cyst or thymolipoma.
(Ref: Dahnert p. 537)

11. e. Pleural effusion
Pleural effusion is the commonest thoracic manifestation of rheumatoid arthritis, much more common in men (M:F = 9:1). It is unilateral in the vast majority of cases. The fluid is an exudate with low sugar content and is often seen in the absence of other pulmonary changes.
(Ref: Dahnert p. 528)

12. a. Mediastinal enlargement
Mediastinal lymph node enlargement is a feature of primary TB. The others are seen with reactivation or fibrocavitary TB. Miliary TB can be seen in any phase with haematogenous dissemination but primary presentation is uncommon.
(Ref: Dahnert p. 539)

13. e. Pulmonary contusion
Pulmonary contusion is the commonest manifestation of blunt trauma and indicates trauma to alveoli with alveolar haemorrhage without significant alveolar disruption. Whilst

plain film changes may not be apparent for up to six hours, CT will demonstrate changes almost immediately post-trauma and signs of resolution can be seen as early as 48 hours. If unresolved, it may progress to ARDS.
(Ref: Kaewlai R *et al.* Multidetector CT of blunt thoracic trauma. *Radiographics* 2008; 28: 1555–1570)

14. c. Bronchial atresia
The case describes bronchial atresia with mucoid impaction. Bronchial atresia is a congenital abnormality that is usually discovered incidentally. It results in local obliteration of the proximal lumen of a segmental bronchus. The apicoposterior segment of the left upper lobe is most commonly affected. Airways distal to the atretic segment continue to produce mucous which can lead to mucoid impaction/mucocoele. The airways distal to the atretic segment also develop normally and are ventilated by collateral air shift. This results in the affected lobe appearing hyperexpanded, oligaemic and hyperlucent.
Congenital lobar emphysema can look similar, however there is usually no mucous plug and patients tend to present early.
(Ref: Dahnert p. 471)

15. e. Left common iliac vein
The presence of the renal veins will be demonstrated on the flush IVC injection, and selective injection into the renal veins is not usually necessary. However, it is mandatory to exclude a double IVC. A second IVC originates from the left iliac vein and can be a cause for failure of the filter despite good positioning.

16. b. Areas of air-space shadowing
Acute extrinsic allergic alveolitis is predominantly a type III hypersensitivity reaction. There is poor correlation between the clinical presentation and the radiological changes. Lymphadenopathy is unusual in the acute phase, but is seen more commonly in recurrent disease. The early changes are mainly in the mid zones, but the fibrosis that develops in chronic extrinsic allergic alveolitis is mainly in the upper zones. In the acute phase, diffuse air-space shadowing or multiple opacities are seen.
(Ref: Dahnert p. 494)

17. c. Renal cell cancer
(Ref: Dahnert p. 515)

18. a. Pleural effusion
Whilst all the above are seen in SLE, pleural effusions are the commonest radiographic abnormality.
(Ref: Grainger & Allison pp. 365–366)

19. c. Melanoma
Whilst most metastases are low on T1-weighted and high on T2-weighted imaging, metastases from melanoma have a high signal on T1-weighted imaging due to the paramagnetic effects of melanin.
(Ref: Wang ZJ *et al.* CT and MR imaging of pericardial disease. *Radiographics* 2003; 23: S167–S180)

20. d. RV/LV diameter ratio
(Ref: Ghaye B *et al.* Can CT pulmonary angiography allow assessment of severity and prognosis in patients presenting with pulmonary embolism? What the radiologist needs to know. *Radiographics* 2006; 26: 23–40)

21. c. Central location
BAC can present in a local form as a mass, usually peripheral, subpleural in location or as diffuse persistent/progressive consolidation in patients with a history of smoking. The area of consolidation is often of low attenuation on CT due to copious mucin production. It is the second most common type of malignancy associated with cavitation.
(Ref: Dahnert p. 473)

22. b. Squamous cell cancer
The case describes a Pancoast tumour for which squamous is the most common cell type.
(Ref: Dahnert p. 476)

23. b. Thick wall
Bronchogenic cyst is the most common intrathoracic foregut duplication cyst. It could have all the above features, but in a mediastinal location, the cyst walls are usually thin. Thick-walled cysts are more likely to be oesophageal.
(Ref: Grainger & Allison p. 252)

24. e. Right middle lobe bronchus
The features described are of an endoluminal lesion causing right middle lobe collapse. A lesion in the bronchus intermedius is likely to cause both middle and lower lobe collapse.
(Ref: Grainger & Allison pp. 318–324)

25. a. Hypointense relative to myocardium on T1-weighted images
The lesion described is a left atrial myxoma which has a heterogenous appearance on most MRI sequences and usually demonstrates varying enhancement following gadolinium injection. This is due to varying amounts of myxomatous tissue, fibrous tissue, blood products and tumour necrosis. The majority of the lesion will be hypointense to myocardium on T1-weighted images. On SSFP images, it is hypointense to blood pool and hyperintense to myocardium. The tumour prolapses through the mitral valve and is best seen on cine-gradient echo imaging with a four-chambered long axis view.
(Ref: Sparrow PJ *et al.* MR imaging of cardiac tumors. *Radiographics* 2005; 25: 1255–1276)

26. b. Perianeurysmal soft-tissue mass
Mycotic aneurysms are usually saccular true aneurysms. Periaortic soft-tissue mass is a common feature seen in up to 48% of cases. Periaortic gas is an uncommon feature. Mural thrombus and calcification are rare features.
(Ref: Lee WK *et al.* Infected (mycotic) aneurysms: spectrum of imaging appearances and management. *Radiographics* 2008; 28: 1853–1868)

27. e. Pseudolipoma
The described feature is a partial volume artefact called pseudolipoma caused by juxtacaval fat above the caudate lobe. It has an association with cirrhosis of liver.

(Ref: Kandpal H *et al.* Imaging the inferior vena cava: a road less traveled. *Radiographics* 2008; 28: 669–689)

28. c. Shift of the previously central trachea to the left

All the other changes are expected changes at this stage following a pneumonectomy. However, contralateral shift of the trachea may be indicative of a post-surgical broncho-pleural fistula.
(Ref: Chae EJ *et al.* Radiographic and CT findings of thoracic complications after pneumonectomy. *Radiographics* 2006; 26: 1449–1467)

29. a. Finger-in-glove opacity

Acute allergic bronchopulmonary aspergillosis is seen as homogeneous, tubular, finger-in-glove areas of increased opacity in a bronchial distribution, usually involving the upper lobes. These shadows are related to plugging of airways by hyphal masses with distal mucoid impaction and can migrate from one region to another on HRCT. Thick-walled cavities and pleural thickening are features of saprophytic aspergillosis. Endobronchial lesion with distal atelectasis is seen mainly in chronic necrotising aspergillosis, whilst tree-in-bud appearance is seen with bronchiolitis in airway invasive aspergillosis.
(Ref: Franquet T *et al.* Spectrum of pulmonary aspergillosis: histologic, clinical, and radiologic findings. *Radiographics* 2001; 21: 825–837)

30. a. Submucosal location

Subserosal fibroids, especially pedunculated ones, may often draw their blood supply from adjacent viscera, which may be a cause of failure of the procedure. They are also associated with a higher incidence of complications. Calcific fibroids are less vascular and may not respond well to embolisation. Bulky and multiple fibroids may need multiple interventions or surgery. Adenomyosis is a known cause for failure of the procedure.
(Refs: Kessel & Robertson ch. 15; Ghai S *et al.* Uterine artery embolization for leiomyomas: pre- and postprocedural evaluation with US. *Radiographics* 2005; 25: 1159–1172)

31. e. Lack of bronchial tapering

Whilst all the above can be seen in patients with bronchiectasis, a lack of progressive tapering of the bronchi is the most sensitive (80%).
(Ref: Dahnert p. 471)

32. d. Calcification

The case describes hydatid disease. Hydatid cyst of the lungs can present as solid ovoid solitary or occasionally multiple lesions on plain films. When the cyst communicates with a bronchial tree, an air fluid level is demonstrated. Several other signs are described. Whilst bilaterality is less likely (up to 20%), calcification is extremely rare (0.7%).
(Ref: Dahnert p. 500)

33. a. Pleural effusion

Pneumocystis carinii is the most common cause of pneumonia at this stage of the disease. Pleural effusions and lymphadenopathy are not features of PCP.
(Ref: Dahnert p. 519)

34. c. Lower zone fibrosis
The case describes neurofibromatosis I, which is associated with lower zone fibrosis and thin-walled bullae, mainly in the upper zones. Apart from the pulmonary changes, skeletal abnormalities involving the ribs and spine and mediastinal masses may also be seen. (Ref Dahnert p. 315)

35. c. A TI of 200 ms would nullify the signal intensity from the normal myocardium
After an initial LV function study, gadolinium is administered and imaging is commenced 100 minutes later in the same spatial location as the preceding LV study. Inversion recovery pulse is used to nullify the signal from the normal myocardium with a TI of approximately 200 ms. The healthy myocardium appears dark, whilst the ischaemic myocardium appears bright. Too short a TI results in loss of signal from both abnormal and normal myocardium, whilst too long a TI would result in loss of contrast. The images are T1-weighted ECG-gated fast gradient echo images.
(Ref: Jackson E *et al.* Ischaemic and non-ischaemic cardiomyopathies – cardiac MRI appearances with delayed enhancement. *Clin Radiol* 2007; 62: 395–403)

36. b. Early myocarditis – patchy, focal subendocardial pattern
In early myocarditis, the enhancement pattern is typically epicardial.
(Ref: Jackson E *et al.* Ischaemic and non-ischaemic cardiomyopathies – cardiac MRI appearances with delayed enhancement. *Clin Radiol* 2007; 62: 395–403)

37. d. Intercostal schwannoma
The description is of a posterior mediastinal lesion obscuring part of the descending thoracic aorta. The other lesions are anterior mediastinal apart from hilar lymphadenopathy, which is hilar/middle mediastinal.
(Ref: Grainger & Allison p. 254)

38. d. High signal on T2-weighted images
PMF has a peripheral location which moves towards the hilum on follow-up imaging. Calcification and cavitation may also be seen. PMF lesions can be FDG-avid on PET-CT. However, high signal in a mass on T2-weighted images is strongly suspicious for malignancy.
(Ref: Chong S *et al.* Pneumoconiosis: comparison of imaging and pathologic findings. *Radiographics* 2006; 26: 59–77)

39. e. Loffler syndrome
This is described as simple eosinophilic pneumonia but is of unknown aetiology. Pathologically, there is interstitial and alveolar oedema. Patients are usually asthmatic/atopic but have mild or no symptoms. Classical chest radiograph appearance is of fleeting infiltrates with transient and shifting peripheral consolidation.
(Ref: Dahnert p. 506)

40. e. Bronchioloalveolar carcinoma
BAC usually presents as a peripheral, subpleural mass or persistent patch of consolidation. All the others can present as endobronchial lesions.
(Ref: Dahnert p. 473)

41. b. To identify the hepatic veins
The hepatic veins do not need to be identified routinely prior to filter insertion. Most filters are deployed in an infrarenal position, unless there is IVC thrombus which would preclude this, in which case the filter is positioned in the suprarenal position. A left iliac injection is performed to rule out a left IVC, which could be a cause of filter failure.
(Ref: Kessel & Robertson ch. 16)

42. b. Multiple bilateral small cysts
Phakomatoses are a group of neurocutaneous syndromes, several of which have other multi-system abnormalities, including intrathoracic findings. These include neurofibromatosis I and II, Sturge–Weber syndrome, von Hippel Lindau syndrome, Osler–Rendu–Weber syndrome and tuberous sclerosis. The above features describe multiple renal angiomyolipomas, which are a feature of tuberous sclerosis. These patients may demonstrate multiple thin-walled cysts with lower zone fibrosis (forme fruste of LAM).
(Ref: Dahnert p. 331)

43. e. Posterior mediastinal lymph nodes
All the above are features of mediastinal lymphadenopathy in sarcoidosis. Whilst sarcoidosis can involve different mediastinal and hilar groups, posterior mediastinal lymphadenopathy is a feature of NHL.
(Ref: Dahnert p. 529)

44. a. Lymphangioleiomyomatosis (LAM)
The cysts in LAM are thin-walled air-containing cysts, rather than cavitation in nodules.
(Refs: Dahnert p. 508; Grant LA *et al.* Cysts, cavities, and honeycombing in multisystem disorders: differential diagnosis and findings on thin-section CT. *Clin Radiol* 2009; 64: 439–448)

45. b. Acute rejection
Hyperacute rejection presents within hours of the transplantation. Reperfusion oedema usually presents within 24 hours of the transplantation, peaking by about day four. Post-transplant infections can be broadly divided into those occurring within the first month (gram-negative bacteria, fungi (candida, aspergillosis)) and those occurring after the first month (CMV, PCP). Anastomotic dehiscence is usually an early feature, but the presentation and features are not those described.
(Ref: Dahnert p. 506)

46. b. Straightening of the right heart border
Left atrial enlargement results in straightening of the left heart border as a result of enlargement of the left atrial appendage. This is especially a feature of rheumatic mitral valve disease.
(Ref: Grainger & Allison pp. 471–472)

47. c. Thickening of a fluid-filled third part of the duodenum
Two weeks post-procedure, all the other features including the presence of ectopic gas may be postoperative. However, presence of a thickened fluid-filled bowel loop would be extremely worrying for an aorto-enteric fistula. Presence of ectopic gas beyond four weeks is much more likely to be abnormal.

(Ref: Vu QD *et al.* Aortoenteric fistulas: CT features and potential mimics. *Radiographics* 2009; 29: 197–209)

48. b. Midaortic syndrome
Midaortic syndrome is a rare vascular abnormality which manifests as narrowing of the abdominal aorta and its branches (including renal arteries – hence hypertension). Its cause is unknown but it is noninflammatory and nonatheromatous. Patients typically present after the age of five years. Diagnosis is made with angiography which reveals smooth, segmental stenoses.

Takayasu arteritis (TA) and neurofibromatosis (NF) are amongst the differentials (the latter can have midabdominal aortic stenosis). However, TA usually affects older patients (12–66 years) and affects females to a much greater degree (M:F = 1:8). Patients with NF and Marfan's would usually have prior medical history. Syphilitic aortitis is rare and typically affects older patients (40–65 year olds).
(Refs: Dahnert p. 655; Pope TL. *Aunt Minnie's Atlas and Imaging-specific Diagnosis*. Edition 2. Philadelphia, PA: Lippincott Williams & Wilkins, 2004)

49. a. Sjogren syndrome
Whilst pulmonary fibrosis is a feature of all the above conditions, bronchiectasis is most likely seen in Sjogren syndrome.
(Ref: Dahnert p. 398)

50. e. Left hilar enlargement
The case describes Swyer–James syndrome (Macleod syndrome). This is a post-infectious constrictive bronchiolitis which causes a small, hyperlucent lung with bronchiectasis and air trapping in expiration. The number and size of pulmonary vessels are also diminished, resulting in a small ipsilateral hilum.
(Ref: Dahnert p. 533)

51. d. Adenoid cystic carcinoma
Adenoid cystic carcinoma is the second most common malignancy of the central airways after squamous cell cancer and often presents as an endoluminal mass with an intact mucosa. Mucoepidermoid carcinoma is rare. Benign tumours are mostly of mesenchymal origin and are rare. Carcinoids in these locations are usually of the typical type.
(Ref: Park CM *et al.* Tumors in the tracheobronchial tree: CT and FDG PET features. *Radiographics* 2009; 29: 55–71)

52. e. Coil embolisation of the aneurysm
This patient was discovered to have an incidental asymptomatic aneurysm. Prophylactic embolisation is generally offered to three groups of patients:

1. Those who have aneurysms greater than 2.5 cm in size.
2. Those with portal hypertension.
3. Those awaiting liver transplantation.

Percutaneous splenic artery aneurysm embolisation using coils is the preferred treatment. Thrombin injection is usually preferred in cases where embolisation has failed. Aneurysms with wider necks often need additional measures such as a detachable balloon.

(Ref: Madoff DC *et al.* Splenic arterial interventions: anatomy, indications, technical considerations, and potential complications. *Radiographics* 2005; 25: S191–S211)

53. c. Axial images are best to assess spinal canal and foraminal involvement

Sagittal and axial images are the most important acquisitions to assess the local extent and involvement of vital neurovascular structures by the tumour, with coronal imaging adding very little further information. T1-weighted images are the most important to assess resectability and should be acquired first. The subclavian vessels can be seen quite clearly as flow voids even without contrast. Gadolinium is usually given to assess for vascular invasion and following adjuvant therapy. Imaging is performed using a neck coil to improve resolution for identifying small local structures.
(Ref: Bruzzi JF *et al.* Imaging of non-small cell lung cancer of the superior sulcus: part 2: initial staging and assessment of resectability and therapeutic response. *Radiographics* 2008; 28: 561–572)

54. a. Urgent cardiothoracic referral

The features described are that of an acute type A intramural haematoma which needs to be treated similarly to that of a Stanford type A aortic dissection and so cardiothoracic surgical opinion is warranted. CT has delineated the extent of the acute intramural haematoma and further imaging would add little. These patients are at increased risk of progressing to a true dissection which carries a high mortality. Whilst endovascular treatment may be considered for selective cases, involvement of the proximal ascending aorta will preclude this.
(Ref: Castaner E *et al.* CT in nontraumatic acute thoracic aortic disease: typical and atypical features and complications. *Radiographics* 2003; 23: S93–S110)

55. e. Multiple stenoses of the mid portion of the renal arteries

In a female patient of this age, fibromuscular dysplasia is the most likely abnormality. Fibromuscular dysplasia involves the mid and distal portions of the renal artery as well as the intrarenal branches, with multiple stenoses and aneurysms revealing a string-of-beads appearance. The ostia and the proximal portion are much less commonly involved. It responds very well to angioplasty, unlike ostial atherosclerotic disease which often needs stenting. Typically it is the medial layer that is affected although all layers can demonstrate changes.
(Refs: Dahnert p. 957; Grainger & Allison p. 841)

56. c. Flow of contrast towards the porta hepatis usually indicates puncture of the biliary tree

Usually the right hepatic vein (RHV) is the preferred route of access to the right portal vein, which lies anterior to the RHV. Flow of contrast towards the porta, and especially if it remains there, usually indicates biliary puncture. Puncture of portal vein and hepatic artery usually result in contrast flowing to the periphery. The shunt gradient should be less than 12 mm of mercury. Stenoses usually tend to occur in the hepatic vein or the shunt itself.
(Ref: Kessel & Robertson ch. 16)

57. b. Aortic injury is the usual cause of mediastinal haematoma

A normal PA chest radiograph has a very high negative predictive value (95–98%) and the absence of a mediastinal haematoma on a non-contrast CT also effectively rules out

the presence of aortic injury. The source of the mediastinal haematoma is usually the azygous, hemiazygous, internal mammary and intercostal vessels. Aortic injury is usually circumferential (85%).
(Ref: Dahnert p. 659)

58. d. Dilated pulmonary veins
This patient has developed Eisenmenger syndrome with reversal of his longstanding left-to-right shunt across the ASD. All of the features listed except dilated pulmonary veins are generally present.
(Ref: Dahnert p. 635)

59. b. Bronchogenic carcinoma
The changes described indicate lymphangitis carcinomatosis. Whilst similar appearances are seen in sarcoidosis, the changes are usually in the upper lobe and pleural effusion is rare. In heart failure, the interlobar septal thickening is usually smooth and usually bilateral. In EAA, pleural effusion is rare and changes are more bronchocentric and bilateral. The polygonal structure is usually distorted in both EAA and cryptogenic fibrosis, where the changes are again subpleural.
(Ref: Dahnert p. 509)

60. c. Field inhomogeneity artefacts are more common on a 3T scanner than a 1.5T scanner
Dark rim artefacts are typically seen on the endocardial aspect on cardiac MR imaging. Spike artefacts are typically sporadic and transient, whilst RF artefacts usually involve all images of the series. At the same bandwidth, image acquisition is quicker with spoiled GRE acquisition. However, often, a lower bandwidth has to be used to improve the signal-to-noise ratio of these sequences and so SSFP imaging may be quicker. In prospective gating, to compensate for physiologic variations in heart rate, the acquisition window is usually 10–20% shorter than the average RR interval, missing out on the end diastole, and hence it is not very useful for assessing diastolic dysfunction.
(Ref: Saremi F *et al.* Optimizing cardiac MR imaging: practical remedies for artefacts. *Radiographics* 2008; 28: 1161–1187)

Musculoskeletal and trauma – Questions

1. A 17 year old girl presents with pain in the distal forearm which has worsened over the last six to eight weeks. Plain films show an eccentric lytic radiolucency in the distal radius with a soap-bubble appearance. The most likely pathology is:
   a. Enchondroma
   b. Aneurysmal bone cyst
   c. Simple bone cyst
   d. Fibrous dysplasia
   e. Chondroblastoma

2. A 35 year old man presents with increasing stiffness in his knee and soft-tissue swelling around the joint. Plain films show multiple areas of irregular cyst-like radiolucencies in the distal femur. There are no areas of abnormal calcification and there is no evidence of periarticular osteoporosis. MR shows a low signal joint effusion on both T1 and T2 sequences. The most likely diagnosis is:
   a. Synovial osteochondromatosis
   b. Pigmented villonodular synovitis
   c. Osteoarthritis
   d. Reiter's syndrome
   e. Osteomyelitis

3. A 56 year old motorcyclist has a trauma series of plain films following a road traffic accident. On evaluation of the lateral cervical spine film, which of the following soft-tissue parameters would be a concerning feature?
   a. Predental space of 3 mm
   b. Nasopharyngeal space of 7 mm
   c. Retropharyngeal space of 10 mm
   d. Retrotracheal space of 20 mm
   e. Decreased disc space at the C5/6 level

4. A 20 year old man presents with an increasingly painful right thigh which is worse at night. Plain films of the area show a lucent area measuring approximately 8–9 mm in the distal femur surrounded by extensive sclerosis. The most likely diagnosis is:
   a. Osteoblastoma
   b. Giant cell tumour
   c. Brodie's abscess
   d. Osteoid osteoma
   e. Chondroblastoma

5. In a 65 year old woman with a fracture of the neck of the humerus, which of the following classification systems to describe the fracture would be useful in guiding the surgical management?
   a. Garden classification
   b. Neer classification
   c. Weber classification
   d. Fryman system
   e. Crosby–Fitzgibbon system

6. A 60 year old woman presents to her GP with renal colic and hypercalcaemia. She has the following findings on plain film: subperiosteal bone resorption of the proximal phalanges of the hands, chondrocalcinosis of the articular cartilage at the knee joints, and a well-defined lytic lesion in the body of the mandible. The most likely unifying diagnosis is:
   a. Parathyroid adenoma
   b. Parathyroid carcinoma
   c. Renal osteodystrophy
   d. Osteomalacia
   e. Myeloma

7. In a 21 year old man with symptoms of chronic back pain, pain in his feet, particularly the great toe and metatarsophalangeal joints, and bilateral sacroiliitis on plain films, the most likely diagnosis is:
   a. Ankylosing spondylitis
   b. Gout
   c. Inflammatory bowel disease-related arthropathy
   d. Reiter's syndrome
   e. Psoriatic arthritis

8. A 45 year old woman falls onto her outstretched hand. The following findings on PA and lateral wrist plain films indicate which pathology? A scapholunate angle of 70°, a capitolunate angle of less than 20°, and a 4 mm gap between scaphoid and lunate on PA view.
   a. Normal appearances
   b. Scapholunate dissociation
   c. Volar intercalated segment instability (VISI)
   d. Dorsal intercalated segment instability (DISI)
   e. Perilunate dislocation

9. A young man presents to A&E following a fall onto his outstretched right arm. Plain films of the right forearm show a fracture of the distal forearm with volar angulation of the distal fragment with no intra-articular component. The carpal bones remain well aligned. Which of the following injuries has he sustained?
   a. Smith's fracture
   b. Barton's fracture
   c. Monteggia fracture
   d. Galeazzi fracture
   e. Colles fracture

10. A 24 year old man injured his left knee whilst skiing. He presents with pain and swelling over the lateral aspect of the knee joint. AP plain radiographs demonstrate an avulsion fracture of the lateral aspect of the proximal tibia below the articular surface. A joint effusion is also seen. The most likely associated ligamentous injury is to which of the following structures?
    a. Posterior cruciate ligament
    b. Anterior cruciate ligament
    c. Medial collateral ligament
    d. Lateral collateral ligament
    e. Ligament of Humphry

11. A 22 year old man presents to his GP with pain in his right knee which is gradually worsening in severity and is relatively resistant to analgesia. MRI of the knee demonstrates an area of geographic bone destruction in the distal femur with a wide zone of transition. There is marked aneurysmal dilatation of the bone and a fluid-fluid level is present within the lesion. The most likely diagnosis is:
    a. Plasmacytoma
    b. Simple bone cyst
    c. Giant cell tumour
    d. Telangiectatic osteosarcoma
    e. Parosteal osteosarcoma

12. A 32 year old footballer sustains an avulsion injury to the anterior superior iliac spine during training. Which of the following muscles is likely to be affected?
    a. Sartorius
    b. Gracilis
    c. Iliopsoas
    d. Rectus femoris
    e. Semimembranosus

13. A middle-aged woman undergoes an MRI of the lumbar spine for longstanding lower back pain. She has no specific neurological signs and is otherwise well. MRI shows some lower lumbar spine facet joint arthropathy and a 2×2 cm well-defined rounded lesion in the L3 vertebral body. This displays high signal on both the T1 and T2 sequences. The most likely explanation for this lesion is:
    a. Discitis
    b. Lymphoma
    c. Myeloma
    d. Metastatic deposit
    e. Haemangioma

14. A 21 year old long-distance runner complains of increasing right groin pain. Plain films show no acute bony injury, but demonstrate a pistol grip deformity of the femoral head, an osseous bump deforming the femoral head–neck junction and an alpha angle of 70°. The acetabulum appears normal. The most likely diagnosis is:
    a. Hip dysplasia
    b. Pincer-type acetabular impingement
    c. Cam-type acetabular impingement

d. Sportsman's hernia

e. Avascular necrosis

15. A 24 year old rugby player attends A&E following a tackle during which he felt his left shoulder dislocate. Initial plain radiographs confirm an anterior inferior dislocation of the left shoulder. Which of the following statements is true?
a. The humeral head lies inferior and lateral to the glenoid on the AP view
b. The presence of a Hill–Sachs defect indicates previous dislocation
c. Hill–Sachs lesions are more common than Bankart lesions
d. Anterior dislocation accounts for 50% of shoulder dislocations
e. A Hill–Sachs lesion affects the inferior aspect of the humeral head

16. In a 26 year old woman with sickle cell disease, which one of the following would not be considered a typical musculoskeletal manifestation of the disease?
a. Osteopaenia and trabecular thinning
b. 'Bone within bone' appearance
c. Avascular necrosis of the femoral head
d. Posterior vertebral scalloping
e. Fish deformity of the vertebrae

17. A 74 year old woman presents with back pain and no history of recent trauma. Lateral plain radiographs show partial collapse of the L2 vertebral body. Which of the following findings would be more suggestive of osteoporotic collapse than malignancy?
a. Complete replacement of the normal marrow signal within the vertebral body on T1 imaging
b. Bilateral pedicular involvement with expansion of the right pedicle
c. Bulging and convex appearance to the vertebral body
d. Nodular irregular epidural mass
e. Intervertebral vacuum phenomenon

18. A 23 year old man sustains a Jefferson fracture to his cervical spine following an injury in which he dived into a shallow swimming pool, hitting his head on the bottom. Which of the following regarding his injury is incorrect?
a. Displacement of the lateral masses of C1 relative to the dens on an odontoid view indicates a transverse ligament rupture
b. Associated C2 fracture will be present in up to 30% of cases
c. Jefferson fractures are usually associated with a neurological deficit
d. Up to 50% are associated with a further cervical spine injury
e. There may be associated vertebral artery injury

19. A 50 year old woman presents with a mass on the plantar aspect of her right foot. Ultrasound reveals a small oval-shaped lesion between the plantar portions of the metatarsal heads. MRI characteristics of the lesion are low-to-intermediate signal on T1 and low signal intensity on T2. Which of the following is the most likely diagnosis?
a. Lipoma
b. Morton's neuroma
c. Plantar fibromatosis

    d. Giant cell tumour of the tendon sheath

    e. Ganglion cyst

20. Following a traumatic left elbow fracture, a young man complains of paraesthesia in his left ring and little fingers. He also starts to notice weakness of his left hand. A diagnosis of ulnar nerve entrapment is made. Which of the following muscles will not be affected?

    a. Abductor digiti minimi

    b. Abductor pollicis brevis

    c. Adductor pollicis

    d. Flexor carpi ulnaris

    e. Flexor digiti minimi

21. A routine pre-operative chest X-ray in a 62 year old woman shows bilateral erosion of the distal clavicles. Which one of the following conditions might be responsible?

    a. Hypoparathyroidism

    b. Rheumatoid arthritis

    c. Langerhans' cell histiocytosis

    d. Ankylosing spondylitis

    e. Sarcoidosis

22. A 74 year old woman with back pain presents to her GP. Initial plain radiographs of her spine show multiple sclerotic metastatic lesions. The most likely primary tumour would be:

    a. Renal cell carcinoma

    b. Melanoma

    c. Bronchial carcinoid

    d. Bladder

    e. Colorectal carcinoma

23. An elderly gentleman complaining of generalised aching in his lower limbs is shown to have bilateral distal tibial periostitis. There is no underlying bone lesion identified. Which of the following would be the most likely explanation?

    a. Arterial insufficiency

    b. Thyroid acropachy

    c. Trauma

    d. Pachydermoperiostosis

    e. Hypertrophic pulmonary osteoarthropathy

24. A 28 year old man is brought into the emergency department following an assault during which he was stabbed in the left flank. He has a 1.3 cm wound just below the left costal margin in the mid-axillary line. No information regarding the knife has been obtained. His renal function is within normal limits and he has no contrast allergies. The optimal CT protocol for scanning his abdomen would include the following contrast:

    a. IV contrast only

    b. Oral contrast and rectal contrast

    c. IV contrast and oral contrast

    d. Oral, rectal and IV contrast

    e. IV contrast and rectal contrast

25. A 75 year old man who is on warfarin for atrial fibrillation is involved in a high-speed road traffic accident in which he sustains a head injury. He lost consciousness at the scene. On arrival at the A&E department his GCS is 15. He has no other obvious injuries. According to NICE guidelines, his management should include the following:
    a. Skull radiograph
    b. No immediate imaging but admission for regular neurological observations
    c. CT head
    d. Skull radiograph followed by CT head
    e. MRI head

26. A young man with limited range of movement at the shoulder joint, a webbed neck and plain film findings of a hypoplastic scapula which is elevated and medially rotated with an associated omovertebral bone is likely to have which associated syndrome?
    a. Turner's syndrome
    b. Down's syndrome
    c. Klippel–Feil syndrome
    d. Neurofibromatosis
    e. Cleidocranial dysostosis

27. A 52 year old woman presents to her GP with a longstanding history of lower back pain which has suddenly worsened in severity over the past few days. An urgent MRI scan of the lumbar spine shows a right paracentral disc protrusion at the L4/L5 level. The disc impinges on the lateral recess at this level. The most likely nerve to be affected is the:
    a. Cauda equina
    b. Lumbar plexus
    c. Right L4
    d. Right L5
    e. Right S1

28. An 18 year old student who fell down two stairs and landed on her left knee attends A&E complaining of generalised knee pain but is able to weight bear. No acute bony injury is demonstrated on plain film, however a pedunculated lesion arising from the femoral metaphysis and extending away from the knee joint is seen. The lesion shows continuity with both the marrow and the cortex. The most likely diagnosis is:
    a. Osteochondroma
    b. Osteoblastoma
    c. Osteoid osteoma
    d. Chondroblastoma
    e. Chondromyxoid fibroma

29. A 70 year old male presents with increasing pain in his right hip over the past month. There is no specific history of trauma. A plain radiograph demonstrates the presence of an incomplete fracture of the femoral neck arising from the lateral (convex) side. What is the most likely underlying abnormality of the femoral neck?
    a. Osteomalacia
    b. Metastasis
    c. Osteoid osteoma
    d. Infection
    e. Paget's disease

30. A 75 year old woman presents with increasing pain in her left hip. She had a total hip replacement eight years ago on this side which has been asymptomatic ever since. Plain radiographs demonstrate a lucent line at the bone cement interface of the femoral component. The likely cause for this is:
    a. Infection
    b. Metastasis
    c. Loosening
    d. Myeloma
    e. Trauma

31. A 17 year old patient complains of lower thoracic back pain. Plain radiographs of the thoraco-lumbar spine show wedging of multiple vertebrae at the thoraco-lumbar junction, multiple limbus vertebrae, an increase in the AP diameter with a reduction in the sagittal height of multiple vertebrae, and multiple endplate defects. What is the unifying diagnosis?
    a. Scheuermann's disease
    b. Ankylosing spondylitis
    c. *Mycobacterium tuberculosis*
    d. Hyperparathyroidism
    e. DISH

32. A 70 year old patient complains of back pain and leg pain after walking 50 metres. Plain radiographs show an anterior slip of L4 relative to L5. The spinous process of L4 is also noted to have moved anterior to the L5 spinous process. What type of spondylolisthesis does this represent?
    a. Traumatic
    b. Degenerative
    c. Spondylolytic
    d. Dysplastic
    e. Pathological

33. A 56 year old male is admitted under the orthopaedic team with increasingly severe lower back pain which started three weeks ago. MRI demonstrates an oedematous L4/5 intervertebral disc, marked loss of disc material and oedematous adjacent endplate changes. There is associated paravertebral inflammatory tissue and a small amount of pus within the residual disc space. The findings are consistent with infective discitis. What is the most likely causative organism?
    a. *Mycobacterium tuberculosis*
    b. *Streptococcus pyogenes*
    c. *Staphylococcus aureus*
    d. *Escherichia coli*
    e. *Salmonella*

34. A 25 year old male is involved in a 60 mph road traffic accident with a head-on collision. He was wearing a seat-belt but his car did not have an air-bag. A screening lateral radiograph of the cervical spine shows the following findings: an angular kyphosis centred at C4/C5, a 1 mm anterior slip of C4 on C5, and widening of the interspinous space posteriorly. What is the likely mechanism for this injury?

a. Lateral compression
b. Flexion
c. Extension
d. Combination
e. Rotation

35. A young man presents to his GP complaining of longstanding back pain. He says he has been diagnosed with a 'syndrome' in the past but cannot remember the details. Which of the following signs is more likely to suggest a diagnosis of homocystinura than Marfan's syndrome?
a. Arachnodactyly
b. Osteoporosis
c. Scoliosis of the spine
d. Autosomal dominant inheritance
e. Upward lens dislocation

36. A 56 year old woman slips off the pavement onto the road and her outstretched foot is run over by a passing car. She has immediate severe midfoot pain. Plain radiographs taken on arrival at the emergency department confirm a Lisfranc fracture dislocation of the midfoot. Which two bones does the Lisfranc ligament attach to?
a. First metatarsal and intermediate cuneiform
b. First metatarsal and medial cuneiform
c. Second metatarsal and medial cuneiform
d. Second metatarsal and intermediate cuneiform
e. First and second metatarsals to the medial and intermediate cuneiforms

37. A 24 year old man suffers a short oblique fracture of his distal tibia from a direct blow during a football game. He is treated with an intramedullary nail with a good reduction being achieved. Fourteen days later the foot becomes very tender, red and swollen but all haematological and biochemical parameters remain normal. Plain radiographs show spotty osteoporosis and subchondral erosions. Which of the following is the most likely diagnosis?
a. Disuse osteoporosis
b. Charcot joints
c. Infection
d. Regional sympathetic dystrophy
e. Rheumatoid arthritis

38. A 25 year old woman attends A&E after falling onto her right hand. A plain film of her hand is taken in order to exclude fracture. No bony injury is seen. On examination, however, there is painless swelling of the right index finger which she says has been present for a few weeks. Incidental note is made of a small central lesion within the medullary cavity of the middle phalanx of the index finger. There is no cortical breakthrough or periosteal reaction but there is bulbous expansion of the bone with thinning of the cortex. The lesion contains dystrophic calcifications. This is most likely to represent:
a. Giant cell tumour of the tendon sheath
b. Unicameral bone cyst
c. Brown tumour

    d. Enchondroma
    e. Epidermal inclusion cyst

39. A 72 year old woman presents to her GP with pain in her right shoulder which is worse on movement. Plain films of the right shoulder show loss of subacromial space and superior subluxation of the humeral head. She is referred for an ultrasound with a suspected supraspinatus tear. Which is the best position of the arm for visualisation of the free edge of the supraspinatous tendon?
    a. Adduction and internal rotation
    b. Abduction and internal rotation
    c. Adduction and external rotation
    d. Abduction and external rotation
    e. Flexion and internal rotation

40. A 57 year old man with increasing pain and stiffness in his hands and feet and worsening back pain presents to his GP. Plain films of his hands show sclerosis of the terminal phalanges and several 'pencil-in-cup' erosions. There is destruction of the interphalangeal joint of his right great toe with exuberant periosteal reaction. There is also erosion of the posterior margin of the calcaneus. The most likely diagnosis is:
    a. Reiter's syndrome
    b. Ankylosing spondylitis
    c. Rheumatoid arthritis
    d. Psoriatic arthritis
    e. Osteoarthritis

41. A 20 year old student complains of a six-week history of pain and tenderness in his right thigh associated with a soft-tissue mass. There is no definite history of trauma. CT of the region shows a mass in the right distal femur with well-defined mineralisation at the periphery and a less distinct lucent centre. On plain film, there is faint calcification within the lesion and a radiolucent zone separating the lesion from bone. The most likely cause is:
    a. Tumoural calcinosis
    b. Osteomyelitis
    c. Myositis ossificans
    d. Parosteal sarcoma
    e. Osteosarcoma

42. A 60 year old man is referred for an MRI of his left upper leg after noticing a slowly enlarging firm mass measuring approximately 7–8 cm in maximum diameter. The mass is located in the quadriceps muscle group and is causing cortical erosion of adjacent bone. There are poorly defined calcifications within it and MR shows a poorly defined lesion which is isointense to muscle on T1-weighted imaging and hyperintense on T2-weighted imaging. The most likely diagnosis is:
    a. Malignant fibrous histiocytoma
    b. Benign fibrous histiocytoma
    c. Liposarcoma
    d. Fibrosarcoma
    e. Elastofibroma

43. A 27 year old man who attends A&E following an alleged assault is shown to have a left-sided longitudinal temporal bone fracture. Which of the following is a correct association?
    a. Facial nerve palsy in 50% of cases
    b. Incudostapedial joint dislocation
    c. Sensorineural hearing loss
    d. Ophthalmoplegia
    e. Rhinorrhoea

44. A 24 year old woman presents with a painless mass on the dorsal aspect of the right index finger measuring approximately 1 × 1 cm. MRI shows a lobulated lesion which has low signal intensity on both T1- and T2-weighted imaging. Which of the following is the most likely diagnosis?
    a. Haemangioma
    b. Lipoma
    c. Ganglion cyst
    d. Giant cell tumour of the tendon sheath
    e. Neurilemmoma

45. A dental radiograph of a 47 year old woman shows loss of the lamina dura of the majority of the teeth. Which of the following would be a possible cause?
    a. Osteopetrosis
    b. Hypoparathyroidism
    c. Scleroderma
    d. Sickle cell anaemia
    e. Myeloma

46. A 28 year old long-distance runner is to undergo MR arthrography of the hip joint for a suspected labral tear. Which of the following statements is correct regarding MR arthrography?
    a. A solution of 20 mmol/L gadopentetate dimeglumine is injected into the hip joint under fluoroscopic guidance
    b. Patients with developmental dysplasia of the hip are at increased risk of labral tears
    c. A communication between the joint capsule and the iliopsoas bursa is always pathological
    d. T2-weighted imaging is used to visualise the high signal of the gadopentetate dimeglumine solution
    e. The normal labrum has uniformly high signal on T1-weighted imaging

47. A 24 year old woman presents with worsening frontal headaches and a sixth nerve palsy. A non-enhanced CT shows a lesion situated within the clivus with associated bony destruction; there is soft-tissue extension into the nasopharynx. MRI shows a large inter-osseous mass which is isointense to brain T1-weighted imaging and hyperintense on T2. The most likely diagnosis is:
    a. Sphenoid sinus cyst
    b. Meningioma
    c. Nasopharyngeal carcinoma
    d. Metastasis
    e. Spheno-occipital chordoma

48. Regarding scaphoid fractures, which of the following statements is correct?
    a. 80% of scaphoid fractures occur at the waist
    b. Approximately 5% of scaphoid fractures are complicated by avascular necrosis
    c. Injury is typically due to hyperextension
    d. Up to 60% of scaphoid fractures cannot be seen on initial radiograph
    e. The specificity of CT in diagnosing scaphoid fractures is 60–70%

49. A 24 year old man is involved in a road traffic accident. On arrival in A&E he is haemodynamically unstable and there is concern regarding pelvic fracture and associated active extravasation. On multidetector CT, which of the following features is more suggestive of pseudoaneurysm than active extravasation?
    a. Ill-defined area of high attenaution on arterial phase imaging
    b. Presence of a haemoperitoneum
    c. Washout of the high-attenuation area on delayed imaging
    d. Layering appearance on delayed imaging
    e. Haemodynamically unstable patient

50. A 27 year old woman is brought into A&E following a road traffic accident in which she was knocked down by a car. On arrival she has a GCS of 15 but is haemodynamically unstable and on examination she has abdominal bruising. The A&E consultant has performed a FAST (focused assessment with sonography in trauma) scan in resus and cannot see evidence of free fluid. What is the approximate minimal detectable fluid volume by FAST scanning?
    a. 10 ml
    b. 50 ml
    c. 100 ml
    d. 200 ml
    e. 500 ml

51. An A&E SHO has asked you to review a paediatric cervical spine plain film which has been performed on a child who has been involved in a road traffic accident. He is unsure as to whether or not the appearances are normal for a paediatric cervical spine film. Which of the following findings is more likely to represent a true cervical spine injury than a normal variant?
    a. Absence of usual cervical lordosis
    b. Widening of the prevertebral soft tissues in expiration
    c. Increased distance between the tips of the C1 and C2 spinous processes in flexion
    d. Wedging of the anterior aspect of the C3 vertebral body
    e. A 7 mm gap between the occipital condyles and the condylar surface of the atlas

52. A 24 year old man has injured his right ankle playing football. The A&E SHO has asked your opinion on the plain radiographs. These show a widening of the medial joint space on the AP ankle view but no evidence of fracture, and an oblique fracture of the proximal shaft of the fibula. This is the typical appearance for which of the following fractures?
    a. Weber B
    b. Maisonneuve
    c. Pilon

   d. Dupuytren's

   e. Fibula stress fracture

53. An 18 year old man undergoes a Tc MDP bone scan to investigate pain in the right hip. A 'hot' lesion is seen in the right proximal femur. No other lesions are seen. Which of the following lesions would appear as 'hot' on a Tc MDP bone scan?
   a. Osteopoikilosis
   b. Fibrous cortical defect
   c. Acute fracture within 12 hours of injury
   d. Fibrous dysplasia
   e. Haemangioma

54. A three month old boy presents with several small painful soft-tissue swellings which have developed over the mandibular region and the right clavicle. Plain films show marked periosteal new bone formation and localised soft-tissue swelling. There is also bone expansion with remodelling of old cortex. The most likely diagnosis is:
   a. Caffey disease
   b. Hypervitaminosis A
   c. Infantile myofibromatosis
   d. Scurvy
   e. Kinky hair syndrome

55. A 29 year old woman presents with a painful right knee which has been worsening over the previous few weeks. A plain film of the right knee shows an oval expansile lesion with a radiolucent centre in the metaphyseal region of the proximal tibia. There is a sclerotic margin and geographic bone destruction. There are internal septations and stippled calcification. There is no periosteal reaction. The most likely diagnosis is:
   a. Non-ossifying fibroma
   b. Chondroblastoma
   c. Giant cell tumour
   d. Chondromyxoid fibroma
   e. Chondrosarcoma

56. A 56 year old woman who has had chronic wrist pain since a fall several months previously is referred for an MR arthrogram of her wrist with a suspected triangular fibrocartilage complex (TFCC) tear. Which of the following would be the best sequence for visualising a TFCC tear?
   a. T1 axial
   b. T2 coronal
   c. Gradient echo sagittal
   d. T2 sagittal
   e. T1 sagittal

57. A 64 year old woman undergoes MRI of her left knee for investigation of chronic knee pain. Which of the following would be considered an abnormal finding on MR?
   a. Bowing of the posterior collateral ligament on sagittal imaging
   b. Low signal ACL on T1-weighted imaging
   c. High signal around the MCL on T2* on coronal imaging

    d. Low signal of the menisci on both T1- and T2-weighted imaging

    e. Medial patellar plica

58. A 53 year old woman attends A&E with a short history of dull right heel pain. She is otherwise fit and well and there is no history of trauma. Plain radiographs of the right foot and ankle reveal a 2 cm expansile non-aggressive lesion in the calcaneum. It has a thin, well-defined sclerotic border. There is no periosteal reaction but there is a small calcified central nidus. The most likely cause of the lesion is:

    a. Aneurysmal bone cyst

    b. Intra-osseous lipoma

    c. Lipoblastoma

    d. Fibrous dysplasia

    e. Desmoplastic fibroma

59. A three-year-old boy attends A&E with a history of a seizure. He has known congenital cardiomyopathy. A chest radiograph shows sclerosis and expansion of several ribs. Previous plain films have shown bone islands within the vertebrae and long bones and bone cysts within the phalanges. Which of the following conditions would be likely to underly these findings?

    a. Down's syndrome

    b. Tuberous sclerosis

    c. Sturge–Weber syndrome

    d. Neurofibromatosis

    e. Sarcoidosis

60. A 27 year old man falls onto his right hand during a game of rugby. He attends the A&E department and a plain film of the right hand shows a comminuted fracture through the base of the thumb metacarpal with an intra-articular component. This is the description of which of the following fractures?

    a. Rolando's fracture

    b. Bennett's fracture

    c. Gamekeeper's thumb

    d. Boxer's fracture

    e. Barton's fracture

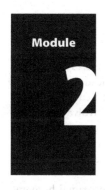

Musculoskeletal
and trauma – Answers

1. b. Aneurysmal bone cyst
Aneurysmal bone cyst is most common in females and 75% occur under 20 years of age. The classic presentation is of pain of relatively acute onset with a rapid increase in severity over 6–12 weeks. Common locations include the spine, with a slight preponderance for the posterior elements, and the metaphysis of long bones – femur, tibia, humerus and fibula. The lesion is usually expansile with thin internal trabeculations giving it the characteristic soap-bubble appearance.
(Ref: Dahnert p. 45)

2. b. Pigmented villonodular synovitis
Pigmented villonodular synovitis is a relatively rare condition which usually presents in the third or fourth decade. It is a monoarticular, painful disease which causes a decreased range of movement at the affected joint. It is most common at the knee (80%) followed by the hip, ankle, shoulder and elbow. Haemorrhagic 'chocolate' effusion is characteristic. Low signal effusion on all sequences at MR is characteristic. There is no calcification or osteoporosis, and joint space narrowing is a late feature.
(Ref: Dahnert pp. 146–147)

3. c. Retropharyngeal space of 10 mm
This is too wide for the retropharyngeal space. The correct acceptable limits for soft-tissue measurements are as follows:
- Predental space 3 mm in adults, 5 mm in children.
- Nasopharyngeal space (anterior to C1) 10 mm.
- Retropharyngeal space (C2–C4) 5–7 mm.
- Retrotracheal space (C5–C7) 22 mm.

Disc spaces should be roughly equal throughout the cervical spine. Narrowing of a disc space is usually due to degenerative change, but widening would be a more concerning feature.
(Ref: Rogers p. 386)

4. d. Osteoid osteoma
This most commonly presents in the second and third decades. The male:female ratio is 2.5:1. Classically it presents with increasing pain which is worse at night and often relieved with aspirin. Spinal lesions often lead to painful scoliosis. Almost any site in the body may be affected but the most common regions are the lower limb and spine.
(Ref: Grainger & Allison pp. 1846–1847)

5. **b. Neer classification**

The Neer classification system is used to grade humeral neck fractures. This system describes four parts – greater tuberosity, lesser tuberosity, humeral head and shaft of humerus. According to Neer, a fracture is displaced if there is more than 1 cm of displacement and 45° angulation between any two segments. Two-part fractures involve any of the four parts and include one fragment that is displaced. Three-part fractures include a displaced fracture of the surgical neck in addition to either a displaced greater tuberosity or lesser tuberosity fracture. Four-part fractures include displaced fractures of the surgical neck and both tuberosities.

(Ref: Mahadeva D *et al.* Reliability of the Neer classification system in proximal humeral fractures: a systematic review of the literature. *Trauma* 2008; **10**: 175–182)

6. **a. Parathyroid adenoma**

Parathyroid adenoma would be the most likely cause of primary hyperparathyroidism. Parathyroid carcinoma would produce a similar radiographic picture but is much less common. Brown tumours are seen in both primary and secondary hyperparathyroidism and are most common in the mandible, ribs and pelvis; they have a variable appearance on MRI and may simulate primary or secondary neoplasms.

(Ref: Grainger & Allison p. 1939)

7. **d. Reiter's syndrome**

Reiter's syndrome is the association of urethritis, conjunctivitis and mucocutaneous lesions. Sacroiliitis is usually bilateral but often persists asymmetrically. There is an association with the HLA B27 antigen. Reiter's has a predeliction for the great toe and metatarsophalangeal joints.

(Ref: Grainger & Allison p. 2011)

8. **b. Scapholunate dissociation**

In scapholunate dissociation the scapholunate angle is >60° and there is a >3 mm gap between the scaphoid and lunate on AP view of the wrist. In VISI, capitolunate angle is increased and there is volar angulation of the lunate. In DISI, both scapholunate and capitolunate angles are increased and there is dorsal angulation of the lunate.

(Ref: Rogers p. 859)

9. **a. Smith's fracture**

This description is of a Smith's fracture. More common is a Colles fracture, which is a fracture of the distal radius with dorsal angulation of the distal fragment. A Monteggia fracture is fracture of the ulnar with dislocation of the radial head. A Galeazzi fracture is a fracture of the radius with dislocation of the distal ulnar. Barton's fracture is a fracture of the distal radius with dislocation of the distal radiocarpal joint.

(Ref: Helms p. 74)

10. **b. Anterior cruciate ligament**

The fracture described is a Segond fracture, originally documented by Dr Paul Segond in 1879 after a series of cadaveric experiments. The Segond fracture occurs most commonly in association with anterior cruciate ligament injuries (75–100%) and medial meniscal injuries. Due to the high rate of associated injuries, a patient who sustains a Segond fracture

will require further imaging, usually by way of MRI, in order to specifically investigate the ligaments and menisci.
(Refs: Brant & Helms p. 1087; Dahnert p. 62)

11. d. Telangiectatic osteosarcoma
With the MRI finding described, the most likely explanation is that the lesion is a telangiectatic osteosarcoma. This is a rare type of osteosarcoma with a mean age at presentation of 20 years. The most common site is around the knee (62%). Fluid-fluid levels are also seen in giant cell tumours and aneurysmal bone cysts.
(Ref: Dahnert p. 144)

12. a. Sartorius
Sartorius has its origin at the anterior superior iliac spine and inserts into the pes anserinus. A sartorius muscle injury can therefore cause an avulsion fracture of the anterior superior iliac spine. Gracilis has its origin at the inferior pubic ramus, and rectus femoris has its origin at the anterior inferior iliac spine.
(Ref: Moore ch. 5)

13. e. Haemangioma
This is most likely to be a benign haemangioma. These are relatively common lesions seen as incidental findings on spinal imaging. High signal on T1 imaging is indicative of the presence of fat within the lesion. All the other conditions would give a low-signal lesion on T1 imaging.
(Ref: Grainger & Allison p. 1048)

14. c. Cam-type acetabular impingement
Femoroacetabular impingement (FAI) occurs as a result of repetitive microtrauma due to an anatomic conflict between the proximal femur and the acetabular rim at the extremes of motion. An osseous bump at the femoral head–neck junction is present in 50% of cam-type FAI and only 33% of pincer-type FAI. An alpha angle of >55° is indicative of cam-type FAI. The alpha angle, drawn on the AP pelvis radiograph, is formed by a line drawn from the centre of the femoral head through the centre of the femoral neck, and a line from the centre of the femoral head to the femoral head–neck junction, found by the point by which the femoral neck diverges from a circle drawn around the femoral head. A normal patient's alpha angle is around 45°, whereas for patients with FAI it may be around 70°.
(Ref: Tannast M *et al.* Femoroacetabular impingement: radiographic diagnosis – what the radiologist should know. *AJR* 2007; **188**: 1540–1552)

15. c. Hill–Sachs lesions are more common than Bankart lesions
A Hill–Sachs lesion affects the postero-superior aspect of the humeral head and whilst it does often indicate a previous dislocation, this is not necessarily the case and it can be present after a single episode. A Bankart lesion affects the inferior glenoid. Almost 95% of all shoulder dislocations are anterior.
(Ref: Brant & Helms pp. 1011–1015)

16. d. Posterior vertebral scalloping
Posterior vertebral scalloping is not a feature. The remainder are all classic features of sickle cell anaemia, along with 'hair-on-end' appearance of the skull due to coarse granular

osteoporosis and widening of the diploe. Osteomyelitis is a feature and is due to salmonella in over 50% of cases.
(Ref: Dahnert p. 162)

17. e. Intervertebral vacuum phenomenon
Intervertebral vacuum phenomenon is highly specific for osteoporotic collapse, although it is not common. The other features are all more suggestive of malignancy than osteoporotic collapse. Pedicular destruction occurs in 50% of cases of malignant collapse but in less than 1% of osteoporotic collapse.
(Ref: Grainger & Allison p. 1088)

18. c. Jefferson fractures are usually associated with a neurological deficit
Jefferson fractures are not usually associated with neurological deficit. Although there may be retropulsion of fragments into the vertebral canal, spinal cord injury is rare due to the large dimensions of the canal at this level. Vertebral artery injury, however, must be considered and if there is concern either CTA or MRA imaging should be considered.
(Ref: Muratsu H *et al.* Cerebellar infarction resulting from vertebral artery occlusion associated with a Jefferson fracture. *J Spinal Disord Tech* 2005; **18**: 293–296)

19. b. Morton's neuroma
The description is that of a Morton's neuroma. This occurs most commonly in the third metatarsal space and less commonly in the second space. There is often an associated metatarsal bursitis which is a high signal on STIR imaging. Ultrasound is usually the first imaging modality; squeezing the metatarsal heads together during scanning will usually make the lesion more prominent.
(Ref: Dahnert p. 122)

20. b. Abductor pollicis brevis
Abductor pollicis brevis is supplied by the median nerve and would therefore not be affected in an ulnar nerve injury. Due to the anatomic location of the ulnar nerve at the elbow, it can often be damaged leading to denervation and paralysis of the muscles supplied by the nerve. This includes the intrinsic muscles of the hand, which can be very debilitating. Injury to the ulnar nerve at the wrist would lead to severe muscle denervation sparing only the opponens pollicis, the superficial head of the flexor pollicis brevis and the lateral two lumbricals.
(Ref: Moore ch. 6)

21. b. Rheumatoid arthritis
Myeloma, hyperparathyroidism, metastases, cleidocranial dysplasia and Gorlin basal cell nevus syndrome all cause absence of the outer end of the clavicle. Destruction of the medial end of the clavicle is caused by metastases, infection, lymphoma, eosinophilic granuloma, rheumatoid arthritis and sarcoma.
(Ref: Dahnert p. 19)

22. c. Bronchial carcinoid
The most likely from the above list is a bronchial carcinoid. In men the most likely cause would be prostate. All the other conditions are more likely to produce lytic metastases than sclerotic.

(Ref: Ashraf MH. Bronchial carcinoid with osteoblastic metastases. *Thorax* 1977; **32**: 509–511)

23. e. Hypertrophic pulmonary osteoarthropathy
The most likely explanation is hypertrophic osteoarthropathy. Thyroid acropachy changes usually occur in the upper limb. Venous stasis is a cause of periostitis rather than arterial insufficiency. Trauma would be unlikely to be bilateral unless there was a specific history. Pachydermoperiostitis is the idiopathic form of hypertrophic osteoarthropathy, it usually presents around adolescence and is usually associated with clubbing.
(Ref: Dahnert p. 106)

24. d. Oral, rectal and IV contrast
A triple contrast technique has been advocated in penetrating trauma where there may be concern regarding small bowel or colon trauma. If no oral or rectal contrast are given then a small bowel or colon injury can easily be missed.
(Ref: Dondelinger ch. 3)

25. c. CT head
According to NICE guidance he should undergo CT head and the investigation should be performed within the hour following referral. The fact he is anticoagulated, over 65 and experienced a loss of consciousness would all be factors in warranting an urgent CT head.
(Ref: National Institute for Health and Clinical Excellence. *Guidelines for the Management of Head Injury.* September 2007. http://guidance.nice.org.uk/CG56)

26. c. Klippel–Feil syndrome
The collective findings described are of a Sprengel deformity of the shoulder. This occurs as a result of failure of descent of the scapula secondary leading to both cosmetic and functional impairment. The male:female ratio is 3:1 and it is associated with Klippel–Feil syndrome, a condition in which there is fusion of vertebral bodies, and renal anomalies.
(Ref: Dahnert p. 165)

27. d. Right L5
The right L5 nerve root is the most likely to be affected as it will be sitting in the right lateral recess at the L4/5 level. The L4 nerve root will be at the exit foramen and therefore if the protrusion affects only the lateral recess then this nerve will already have exited and therefore not be affected.
(Ref: Moore ch. 4)

28. a. Osteochondroma
The description is classic for an osteochondroma or osteocartilagenous exostosis. These lesions are the most common benign growths of the skeleton, are usually found incidentally and are usually asymptomatic unless complications arise. Complications include fracture, vascular compromise, bursa formation and malignant transformation into chondrosarcoma.
(Ref: Chapman & Nakielny 2003 p. 584)

41

29. e. Paget's disease
Incremental fractures (banana fracture) along the convex side of the bone are classically associated with Paget's disease. These most commonly occur in the femur where they cause lateral bowing, and the tibia where they cause anterior bowing. Compression fractures of the vertebrae are also associated with Paget's.
(Ref: Dahnert p. 144)

30. c. Loosening
Early changes (less than six months) are almost always due to infection. Up to four years, infection remains the most likely cause, but after this point loosening becomes more common. Every year, 38 000 hips are replaced in the UK. A routine postoperative film is usually performed; an excessively varus stem may lead to loosening.
(Ref: Ostlere S, Soin S. Imaging of prosthetic joints. *Imaging* 2003; **15**: 270–285)

31. a. Scheuermann's disease
These are the classical appearances of Scheuermann's disease. This condition usually presents at puberty and consists of vertebral wedging, endplate irregularity and narrowing of the intervertebral disc spaces. The most common location is in the lower thoracic and upper lumbar spine. Schmorl's nodes are often present.
(Ref: Dahnert p. 223)

32. b. Degenerative
This is the classical description of the symptoms and radiology of a degenerative spondylolisthesis. Degenerative spondylolisthesis is usually symptomatic due to spinal stenosis and narrowing of neural foramen. This most commonly occurs at the L4/5 level. Spondylolisis is a defect in the pars interarticularis between superior and inferior articulating processes.
(Ref: Grainger & Allison p. 1377)

33. c. *Staphylococcus aureus*
The most common cause of infective discitis is *Staphylococcus aureus,* which gives the above typical findings. The only other relatively common cause is *Mycobacterium tuberculosis,* which typically spares the disc until late and usually has a large amount of associated pus.
(Ref: Dahnert p. 205)

34. b. Flexion
This describes the typical appearance for a flexion injury as well as the typical mechanism. This would represent a potentially unstable fracture and immobilisation would be essential until further management decisions are made. Flexion teardrop injuries are more common in the lower cervical spine and extension teardrop injuries are more common in the upper cervical spine.
(Ref: Rogers p. 378)

35. b. Osteoporosis
Osteoporosis is a feature of homocystinuria and occurs in 75% of cases, often causing bowing and fracture of the long bones. The other features are all more suggestive of Marfan's syndrome. Although arachnodactyly does occur in homocystinuria (in 30%

of cases), it occurs in 100% of people with Marfan's syndrome. Homocystinuria has an autosomal recessive mode of inheritance.
(Ref: Dahnert p. 103)

36. c. Second metatarsal and medial cuneiform
The Lisfranc ligament attaches between the second metatarsal and medial cuneiform, which is why an injury to this ligament allows the second to fifth metatarsals to drift laterally once they have lost this stabilisation. This is therefore an unstable injury and requires rapid immobilisation. This is a vital injury to detect as long-term sequelae will often result from a delayed diagnosis.
(Ref: Peicha G *et al.* The anatomy of the joint as a risk factor for Lisfranc dislocation and fracture-dislocation. *J Bone Joint Surg Br* 2002; **84**: 981–985)

37. d. Regional sympathetic dystrophy
This is the typical appearance, history and imaging findings for regional sympathetic dystrophy. This may occur following fractures or secondary to other pathologies such as primary or secondary bone tumours. There is overactivity of the sympathetic nervous system causing pain, swelling and hyperaemia with excessive bone resorption. This is usually in a periarticular distribution and may simulate other disease processes.
(Ref: Grainger & Allison p. 1953)

38. d. Enchondroma
This lesion is most likely to be an enchondroma. This is a benign cartilaginous growth in the medullary cavity and is usually asymptomatic. It most commonly occurs in the small bones of the hands and wrist but may also occur in the proximal humerus and proximal femur. Epidermoid inclusion cysts are usually in the distal phalangeal tuft and there is often a history of trauma. A bone cyst would be unusual in the phalanges.
(Ref: Dahnert p. 73)

39. a. Adduction and internal rotation
The best position for visualising the supraspinatous tendon is with the patient's arm in adduction and internal rotation. Often the patient may be asked to place the back of their hand onto their back, or alternatively asking them to simulate putting the hand into the back pocket of their trousers. The most medial part of the tendon when imaged transversely is the free edge – this is where the majority of supraspinatous tears occur.
(Ref: Seibold C *et al.* Rotator cuff: evaluation with US and MR imaging. *Radiographics* 1999; **19**: 685–705)

40. d. Psoriatic arthritis
This is usually HLA B27 positive and is associated with skin and nail changes in the majority of cases. The hands are often described as having sausage digits, and erosions with ill-defined margins are characteristic. Sacroiliitis is often present and most often bilateral. Within the axial skeleton, there is often large bulky vertically orientated soft-tissue ossification giving a 'floating' osteophyte appearance.
(Ref: Dahnert p. 149)

41. c. Myositis ossificans
Often there is no distinct history of trauma, although this is the most common cause. It usually occurs in the large muscles of the extremities and in the early stages it can be difficult to distinguish from soft-tissue sarcomas. It is, however, separate from bone, unlike parosteal sarcoma and post-traumatic periostitis. This is a self-limiting condition, most commonly occurring in young athletic adults, with resorption occurring in approximately one year.
(Ref: Dahnert p. 126)

42. a. Malignant fibrous histiocytoma
Soft-tissue malignant fibrous histiocytoma is the most common primary malignant soft-tissue tumour of later adulthood. It is most commonly seen in the lower extremities. It has a metastatic rate of 42% and most commonly metastasises to the lung. Osseous malignant fibrous histiocytoma presents as a painful, tender, rapidly enlarging mass and most commonly arises in the metaphysis of long bones.
(Ref: Dahnert p. 81)

43. b. Incudostapedial joint dislocation
Longitudinal fractures of the temporal bone are more common than transverse fractures and account for over 85% of temporal bone fractures. They are associated with otorrhea, conductive hearing loss, pneumocephalus, herniation of the temporal lobe and incudostapedial dislocation. Transverse fractures are associated with sensorineural hearing loss, and a higher percentage of facial nerve palsies.
(Ref: Dahnert p. 209)

44. d. Giant cell tumour of the tendon sheath
This is a benign lesion thought to represent an extra-articular form of pigmented villo-nodular hyperplasia. This is low signal on both T1- and T2-weighted imaging due to haemosiderin deposition. It most commonly affects the fingers and characteristically lies along a tendon sheath.
(Ref: Dahnert p. 129)

45. c. Scleroderma
The other causes of loss of the lamina dura include Cushing's disease, Paget's, hyperparathyroidism, osteoporosis, osteomalacia, leukaemia, metastases and Langerhans' cell histiocytosis. Both osteopetrosis and hypoparathyroidism cause thickening of the lamina dura of the teeth.
(Ref: Chapman & Nakielny 2003 p. 391)

46. b. Patients with developmental dysplasia of the hip are at increased risk of labral tears
The increased risk of labral tears in developmental dysplasia is due to the increased stress placed upon the acetabular rim and labrum. A communication between the joint capsule and iliopsoas bursa has been described as a normal finding in 10–15% of patients. A dilute solution of 0.2 mmol/L gadopentetate dimeglumine solution would usually be used for arthrography. A normal labrum has uniformly low signal on T1-weighted imaging with

slightly increased signal on gradient echo imaging. Appearances on T2-weighted imaging can be more variable.
(Ref: Petersilge CA. Chronic adult hip pain: MR arthrography of the hip. *Radiographics* 2000; **20**: S43–S52)

47. e. Spheno-occipital chordoma
The most likely cause is a spheno-occipital chordoma. This is associated with bony destruction in 90% of cases and is most usually within the clivus. Other sites include the sella, petrous temporal bone, floor of middle cranial fossa and jugular fossa. Sacrococcygeal chordoma is the most common subtype of chordoma and is usually located with the fourth or fifth sacral segments. Vertebral/spinal chordoma accounts for only 15–20% of all chordomas and is most often situated in the cervical spine.
(Ref: Dahnert p. 201)

48. c. Injury is typically due to hyperextension
The scaphoid bone is the most commonly fractured carpal bone and the mechanism is usually a fall onto the outstretched hand – ie. hyperextension of the wrist. The reported sensitivities and specificities of CT are 89–97% and 85–100%, respectively. The high negative predictive value of CT (96.8–99%) makes it very useful for ruling out a fracture. Scaphoid fractures are missed on initial radiographs in up to 30% of cases.
(Ref: Kaewlai R *et al*. Multidetector CT of carpal injuries: anatomy, fractures, and fracture-dislocations. *Radiographics* 2008; **28**: 1771–1784)

49. c. Washout of the high-attenuation area on delayed imaging
Washout of the high-attenuation area is one of the features of a pseudoaneurysm. A pseudoaneurysm is likely to be adjacent to a vessel and whilst there will be a relatively well-defined area of high attenuation on arterial phase imaging, this will diminish in intensity on five-minute delayed imaging. In contrast to this, an area of active extravasation will often appear as a jet of high attenuation which continues to collect and enlarge on delayed phase imaging.
(Ref: Hamilton JD *et al*. Multidetector CT evaluation of active extravasation in blunt abdominal and pelvic trauma. *Radiographics* 2008; **28**: 1603–1616)

50. d. 200 ml
The approximate minimal detectable fluid volume is 200 ml. The distribution of free fluid will be determined by both anatomical and physiologic factors and therefore the sensitivity of the scan will depend upon the areas scanned. Ultrasound is often used in conjunction with multidetector CT, particularly in the management of patients who have been involved in trauma.
(Refs: Korner M *et al*. Current role of emergency US in patients with major trauma. *Radiographics* 2008; **28**: 225–244)

51. e. A 7 mm gap between the occipital condyles and the condylar surface of the atlas
This is highly suggestive of craniocervical injury; these injuries are often fatal and are often caused by sudden deceleration. Radiologic evaluation of this injury can be difficult but is crucial in determining further management. The remainder of the findings above can all be

normal variants in the paediatric cervical spine and therefore should be interpreted with care.
(Ref: Lustrin E *et al.* Paediatric cervical spine: normal anatomy, variants and trauma. *Radiographics* 2003; **23**: 539–560)

52. b. Maisonneuve

This is the description of a Maisonneuve fracture (sometimes classified as Weber C3). This injury is often overlooked as the patient may complain only of ankle pain and hence a full tibia/fibula plain film is not taken. This fracture is often associated with ligamentous injury at the ankle, most usually of the anterior talofibular ligament and the postero-inferior talofibular ligament.
(Ref: Rogers p. 1270)

53. d. Fibrous dysplasia

The most common site of monostotic fibrous dysplasia is the ribs, followed by proximal femur and craniofacial bones. Three-quarters of cases present before age 30. Other benign lesions causing a 'hot' on bone scan include Paget's disease, brown tumours, aneurysmal bone cysts, osteoid osteoma and chondroblastoma.

Acute fractures are not usually 'hot' until after the first 24–48 hours.
(Ref: Dahnert p. 79)

54. a. Caffey disease

The most likely diagnosis is Caffey disease. This is a relatively rare self-limiting condition which usually presents before six months of age. The mandible is the most common site and accounts for 80% of cases, followed by the clavicle and the upper limb bones.
(Ref: Dahnert p. 108)

55. d. Chondromyxoid fibroma

This is most commonly seen in the second and third decades and the most common site is the long bones, most often the proximal tibia and distal femur. Non-ossifying fibroma is usually asymptomatic. The appearances of a chondroblastoma would be similar but this would most likely be epiphyseal in location and usually presents in a slightly younger age group.
(Ref: Dahnert pp. 57–58)

56. b. T2 coronal

The best sequence would be a T2 or T2* image for detecting a tear. This is also a useful plane in which to assess for ulnar variance; positive ulnar variance has an association with perforations. The central portion of the articular disc is not well vascularised and therefore a tear in this portion will heal poorly. The peripheral portion, however, has been vascularised.
(Ref: Grainger & Allison pp. 1148–1149)

57. c. High signal around the MCL on T2* on coronal imaging

The only abnormal finding is the presence of high signal around the MCL on T2* imaging. This would represent oedema or haemorrhage around the MCL and may be associated with a tear. Bowing of the PCL occurs when the knee is extended. A medial patellar plica is

a normal finding in approximately 50% of the population. This is an embryological remnant from when the knee was divided into three compartments.
(Ref: Brant & Helms p. 1083)

58. b. Intra-osseous lipoma
The calcaneum is a common location for an intra-osseous lipoma. They do, however, also occur in the extremities, skull and mandible. There is no periosteal reaction unless there is an associated fracture. Imaging features would be similar to those of a unicameral bone cyst. They are often asymptomatic but can present with localised bone pain.
(Ref: Dahnert p. 113)

59. b. Tuberous sclerosis
This is a multi-system autosomal dominant disorder affecting the central nervous system, kidneys, lung and heart. The classic triad of facial angiofibroma, epileptic seizures and mental retardation is only seen in approximately 30% of patients. Skeletal abnormalities include sclerotic calvarial patches or 'bone islands', thickening of diploe, expansion and sclerosis of ribs and periosteal thickening of long bones. Gracile ribs are often seen in association with Down's syndrome.
(Ref: Dahnert p. 331)

60. a. Rolando's fracture
This is the classic description of a Rolando's fracture. A Bennett's fracture is also a fracture of the base of the first metacarpal but with no comminution; this fracture is often less stable than a Rolando's fracture and more often requires surgical fixation. A 'gamekeeper's thumb' often occurs as the result of forced abduction of the thumb and results in disruption of the ulnar collateral ligament.
(Ref: Grainger & Allison p. 1000)

Gastro-intestinal – Questions

1. A 71 year old female with scleroderma undergoes a barium swallow examination. Which one of the following findings concerning the oesophagus would not be consistent with this diagnosis?
   a. Oesophageal dilatation
   b. Superficial ulcers
   c. Hypoperistalsis in the upper third of the oesophagus
   d. Stricture 5 cm above the gastro-oesophageal junction
   e. Oesophageal shortening

2. A 32 year old male front seat passenger is involved in a road traffic accident and sustains blunt abdominal trauma. He is admitted via the emergency department and CT reveals a splenic laceration with subcapsular haematoma. Which one of the following associated injuries is most likely to be found?
   a. Diaphragmatic rupture
   b. Injury to the liver
   c. Injury to the left kidney
   d. Ipsilateral rib fractures
   e. Injury to the small bowel mesentery

3. A neonate is diagnosed with congenital tracheoesophageal (TE) fistula. A plain film demonstrates a gasless abdomen. Which type of TE fistula is associated with this finding?
   a. Type B
   b. Type C
   c. Type D
   d. Type E
   e. None of the above

4. A 60 year old female has a plain abdominal film which shows a grossly distended segment of bowel. Which one of the following features makes a diagnosis of caecal volvulus more likely than sigmoid volvulus?
   a. Pelvic overlap sign
   b. Apex lying above the level of T10
   c. Liver overlap sign
   d. Coffee bean sign
   e. Presence of haustral markings

5. A 40 year old man is admitted to the surgical ward with acute abdominal pain and subsequently a CT abdomen and pelvis is requested. The findings include a 3 cm oval

Module 3 – Gastro-intestinal

mass with central fat density adjacent to the sigmoid colon and with associated fat stranding. Which one of the following is the most likely diagnosis?

a. Diverticulitis
b. Epiploic appendagitis
c. Mesenteric lymphadenitis
d. Meckel's diverticulitis
e. Infected enteric duplication cyst

6. A seven year old boy on chemotherapy for acute leukaemia develops severe right iliac fossa pain and diarrhoea. CT shows ascending colon and caecal wall thickening, with inflammation extending to involve the appendix and terminal ileum and fat stranding in the adjacent mesentery. The most likely diagnosis is:

a. Typhlitis
b. Crohn's disease
c. Acute appendicitis
d. Necrotising enterocolitis
e. Acute leukaemic infiltration

7. A young patient is diagnosed with multiple endocrine neoplasia (MEN) type 3 (also known as type 2b) after an episode of bowel obstruction. Which one of the following features would he be unlikely to have or develop in the future with this diagnosis?

a. Medullary carcinoma of the thyroid
b. Marfanoid appearance
c. Mucosal neuromas of the small bowel
d. Facial angiofibromas
e. Prognathism

8. A 48 year old woman with upper abdominal pain is found to have a 4 cm hypervascular lesion in the head of the pancreas on contrast-enhanced CT. She subsequently has an MR scan; the lesion is of low intensity on fat-saturated T1-weighted and high intensity on T2-weighted imaging. Which of the following is the most likely diagnosis?

a. Pancreatic adenocarcinoma
b. Gastrinoma
c. Insulinoma
d. Macrocystic adenoma
e. Pancreatic pseudocyst

9. An 83 year old woman is investigated for weight loss, and undergoes contrast-enhanced CT scan of the chest, abdomen and pelvis. Multiple hypervascular metastases are found in the liver. Which one of the following is most likely to be the primary tumour?

a. Adenocarcinoma of the stomach
b. Invasive ductal carcinoma of the breast
c. Carcinoid tumour
d. Adenocarcinoma of the sigmoid
e. Pancreatic ductal adenocarcinoma

10. A 32 year old male is referred for a barium swallow by his GP due to dysphagia resistant to medical treatment. A smooth, lobulated, eccentric mass is seen in the middle third of the oesophagus containing foci of calcification. The diagnosis is most likely to be which one of the following?
    a. Leiomyoma
    b. Squamous cell carcinoma
    c. Adenocarcinoma
    d. Oesophageal web
    e. Intramural pseudodiverticulosis

11. A 56 year old woman is diagnosed with pancreatic adenocarcinoma. Which one of the following features on the pancreatic MR contraindicates curative surgery?
    a. Splenic vein invasion
    b. Tumour size of 2 cm
    c. Portal vein invasion
    d. Hepatic artery invasion
    e. Invasion of the second part of the duodenum

12. A 67 year old man is referred for a barium swallow from the surgical outpatient department with a history of dysphagia to solids. A mid-oesophageal stricture is demonstrated. Which one of the following causes is unlikely to be in the differential?
    a. Barrett's oesophagus
    b. Squamous cell carcinoma of the oesophagus
    c. Schatzki ring
    d. Caustic substance ingestion
    e. Epidermolysis bullosa

13. A 71 year old man is referred to CT for unexplained abdominal distension. Low-attenuation intraperitoneal collections with enhancing septae are demonstrated. There is scalloping of the liver border and omental thickening. Which one of the following is most likely to be the underlying cause?
    a. Carcinoid tumour of the appendix
    b. Cystadenocarcinoma of the appendix
    c. Melanosis coli
    d. Mastocytosis
    e. Retroperitoneal fibrosis

14. A 78 year old previously well female is admitted with acute abdominal pain and diarrhoea. Contrast-enhanced CT of the abdomen and pelvis shows thickening of a 13 cm segment of proximal descending colon and mucosal hyperenhancement. The rest of the colon is normal, and the small bowel is unaffected. There is a small amount of free fluid in the pelvis. Which one of the following diagnoses is most likely?
    a. Crohn's colitis
    b. Ulcerative colitis
    c. Ischaemic colitis
    d. Infectious colitis
    e. Pseudomembranous colitis

15. A 27 year old male has recurrent admissions for intermittent low-grade small bowel obstruction of unknown cause. Which one of the following investigations would be most appropriate?
    a. Contrast-enhanced CT abdomen and pelvis
    b. Barium meal
    c. Small bowel enteroclysis
    d. Serial abdominal plain films
    e. Barium follow-through

16. An asymptomatic 46 year old woman has an MR liver following an incidental finding of a focal mass in the right lobe of the liver on ultrasound. The MR shows an 8 cm isolated lesion. It is high signal on T1-weighted sequences and isointense on T2-weighted sequences relative to the normal liver parenchyma. The lesion is most likely to be which one of the following?
    a. Hepatocellular carcinoma
    b. Liver metastasis
    c. Haemangioma
    d. Fibronodular hyperplasia
    e. Adenoma

17. A 26 year old female has an ultrasound scan for right upper quadrant pain and a heterogenous 5 cm solitary liver lesion with central calcifications, and a hyperechoic scar is seen. Blood tests reveal a negative alpha-fetoprotein. MR shows the lesion is hypointense on T1 and hyperintense on T2-weighted imaging. The central scar is hypointense on both sequences. Which of the following diagnoses is most likely?
    a. Hepatic lymphoma
    b. Hepatocellular carcinoma
    c. Fibrolamellar carcinoma
    d. Hepatoblastoma
    e. Hepatic angiosarcoma

18. A 72 year old woman has a pancreatic MR to investigate recurrent episodes of pancreatitis. There is generalised pancreatic atrophy with dilatation of the main pancreatic duct and branch ducts, particularly in the tail. No focal lesion or intraductal calculi are present. Which one of the following diagnoses is most likely?
    a. Microcystic cystadenoma
    b. Intraductal papillary mucinous tumour of the pancreas
    c. Cystic metastases
    d. Cystic islet cell tumour
    e. Pancreatic lipomatosis

19. A 25 year old male presents with abdominal cramps and pain with rectal bleeding. Colonoscopy is normal. CT enteroclysis is performed as part of the investigation, which reveals multiple sessile polyps throughout the jejunum and ileum. Subsequent biopsies reveal these polyps to be hamartomas. Which one of the following syndromes is he most likely to be diagnosed with?
    a. Peutz–Jeghers
    b. Cowden's
    c. Turcot's

    d. Familial polyposis

    e. Gardner's

20. A 17 year old female undergoes screening colonoscopy and is found to have multiple adenomatous polyps throughout the colon. OGD and biopsy reveal multiple hamartomas of the stomach and duodenum. She subsequently has investigation for a painful jaw that reveals a 1 cm round, discrete, dense lesion in the mandible. Which one of the following syndromes is the most likely underlying diagnosis?

    a. Lynch syndrome

    b. Cronkhite–Canada syndrome

    c. Familial adenomatous polyposis

    d. Gardner's syndrome

    e. Peutz–Jegher syndrome

21. A 58 year old male has a CT staging scan following a diagnosis of adenocarcinoma of the body of the pancreas. The tumour is 3 cm in size and extends beyond the boundaries of the pancreas but does not invade any vessels or adjacent organs. Two 1 cm lymph nodes lie adjacent to the tumour. No other nodes, or metastatic disease in the chest, abdomen or pelvis, are identified. The tumour is best staged as which one of the following?

    a. T1N0M0

    b. T1N1M0

    c. T2N0M0

    d. T3N0M0

    e. T3N1M0

22. A 41 year old woman has an outpatient ultrasound scan for intermittent right upper quadrant pain. Five 5 mm gallstones and sludge are present. In addition, there is wall thickening of the gallbladder fundus with multiple foci of increased echogenicity within the wall, each associated with bright artefacts deep to them. Which one of the following is the most likely diagnosis?

    a. Porcelain gallbladder

    b. Emphysematous cholecystitis

    c. Acute cholecystitis

    d. Adenomyomatosis of the gallbladder

    e. Gallbladder carcinoma

23. A 32 year old man has an ultrasound scan for obstructive jaundice. Areas of intrahepatic duct dilatation are seen, with increased echogenicity of the portal triads. ERCP reveals alternating segments of dilatation and stenosis of both the intra- and extrahepatic ducts. Which one of the following diagnoses is most likely?

    a. Primary sclerosing cholangitis

    b. Primary biliary sclerosis

    c. Ascending cholangitis

    d. Choledochal cyst

    e. Congenital hepatic fibrosis

24. A neonate is investigated for obstructive jaundice and as part of the investigation has a hepatobiliary iminodiacetic acid (HIDA) nuclear medicine scan. This shows

a photopaenic area within the liver and lack of visualisation of the small bowel. Which one of the following conditions would be most consistent with these findings?
a. Enteric duplication cyst
b. Biliary duct atresia
c. Choledochal cyst
d. Pancreatic pseudocyst
e. Hepatic cyst

25. A one year old boy is admitted unwell with generalised abdominal tenderness and guarding. A supine plain abdominal film is requested, which shows a large oval radiolucency in the middle of the abdomen, with a well-defined linear opacity in the right upper quadrant. Which one of the following conditions would best explain these appearances?
a. Enteric duplication cyst
b. Choledocal cyst
c. Pneumoperitoneum
d. Duodenal atresia
e. Caecal volvulus

26. A 50 year old male is admitted with epigastric pain, diarrhoea and vomiting. Ascites is present clinically. Serum albumin is low and the patient is anaemic. Colonoscopy is normal but the patient is intolerant of upper gastro-intestinal endoscopy. Barium meal reveals a normal antrum but elsewhere there are diffusely thickened and enlarged gastric folds despite good gastric distension. Which one of the following is the most likely diagnosis?
a. Gastric lymphoma
b. Menetrier's disease
c. Gastric adenocarcinoma
d. Acute gastritis
e. Linitis plastica

27. A 31 year old male is investigated as an outpatient for diarrhoea. A small bowel meal study reveals jejunal dilatation with thickened valvulae conniventes. In the ileum an increased number of mucosal folds are seen. Which of the following diagnoses is most likely?
a. Lymphoma
b. Crohn's disease
c. Coeliac disease
d. Whipple disease
e. Behcet syndrome

28. A 53 year old male is investigated for recurrent episodes of biliary colic. Blood tests reveal eosinophilia and normal liver function tests. Abdominal ultrasound demonstrates a 7 cm cystic structure with a thin hyperechoic wall and several smaller satellite cysts up to 2 cm adjacent to the lesion. Which one of the following diagnoses is most likely?
a. Hydatid cyst
b. Pyogenic abscess
c. Amoebic abscess

    d. Schistosomiasis

    e. Hepatocellular carcinoma

29. A 71 year old female is admitted via A&E with abdominal pain, abdominal distension and vomiting. Plain abdominal film shows multiple dilated loops of small bowel. In addition there is gas projected over the liver shadow which is prominent centrally and has a branching appearance. Gas is not visible over the periphery of the liver. No other abnormality is seen on the plain film. Which of the following diagnoses is most likely?

    a. Small bowel perforation

    b. Small bowel infarction

    c. Gallstone ileus

    d. Emphysematous cholecystitis

    e. Pneumatosis intestinalis

30. A 35 year old male with known ulcerative colitis presents to A&E with severe abdominal pain, pyrexia and diarrhoea. There is no peritonism. Toxic megacolon is suspected clinically. Which one of the following is the most appropriate as first line imaging?

    a. CT

    b. Plain abdominal film

    c. Double contrast barium enema

    d. Single contrast water-soluble enema

    e. Targeted bowel ultrasound

31. As part of an investigation for altered bowel habit, a 32 year old female has a double contrast barium enema performed. Findings include deep and superficial aphthous ulceration from the caecum proximally to the sigmoid colon and the presence of pseudodiverticula. Which one of the following is most likely?

    a. Crohn's disease

    b. Ulcerative colitis

    c. Tuberculosis

    d. Yersinia

    e. Lymphoma

32. A 38 year old patient with AIDS presents with diarrhoea and steatorrhoea. As part of the work-up, small bowel enteroclysis shows thickened jejunal folds with nodularity and evidence of marked jejunal spasm. The ileum has normal appearances. Which one of the following is the most likely underlying cause?

    a. *Cytomegalovirus*

    b. Tuberculosis

    c. *Mycobacterium avium intracellulare*

    d. *Cryptosporidium*

    e. Giardiasis

33. An 81 year old man is investigated for anaemia of unknown cause. He has a barium enema as an outpatient that is reported as normal, but is subsequently admitted with a large gastro-intestinal bleed. Initial upper gastro-intestinal endoscopy is normal. He is haemodynamically unstable and therefore has a mesenteric angiogram, which shows

early opacification and slow emptying of the ileocolic vein. Which one of the following diagnoses is most likely?
a. Angiodysplasia
b. Diverticulosis
c. Meckel's diverticulum
d. Adenomatous polyp
e. Radiation enteritis

34. A 37 year old female has a pelvic MRI for investigation of rectal pain and bleeding, following a normal flexible sigmoidoscopy. This shows a thin-walled dumbbell-shaped 7 cm multilocular cyst. It is in contact anteriorly to the rectum and posteriorly to the presacral fascia, but contained within the mesorectal fascia. Although the rectum is distorted by the mass, the rectum and sigmoid are normal. What is the most likely diagnosis?
a. Rectal duplication cyst
b. Anterior sacral meningocoele
c. Mucinous rectal carcinoma
d. Presacral dermoid
e. Tailgut cyst

35. A 34 year old female is investigated for intermittent abdominal pain and malabsorption. Small bowel meal shows dilatation of the proximal small bowel loops but a normal mucosal fold pattern. Which one of the following is the most likely underlying diagnosis?
a. Coeliac disease
b. Amyloid
c. Whipple disease
d. Giardiasis
e. Eosinophilic gastroenteritis

36. A six week old child has an ultrasound scan of the abdomen performed for non-bilious projectile vomiting. Which one of the following features would support a diagnosis of infantile pylorospasm over a diagnosis of hypertrophic pyloric stenosis?
a. Pyloric muscle wall thickness of 2 mm
b. Pyloric canal length of 19 mm
c. Target sign
d. Antral nipple sign
e. Transverse pyloric diameter of 14 mm

37. A 52 year old male has an unenhanced CT KUB for left renal colic. No cause for the pain is discovered on the CT, however the liver is found to be of increased density relative to the spleen. Which one of the following would be most likely to explain this incidental finding?
a. Excess alcohol intake
b. Amiodarone use
c. Diabetes
d. Steroids
e. Past history of chemotherapy

38. A 68 year old female has a pancreatic MR for characterisation of an isolated lesion within the pancreas seen initially on CT performed for unexplained weight loss. The lesion is 3 cm in diameter, isointense on T1, isointense on T2 STIR and hypointense to pancreatic parenchyma during the arterial phase of gadolinium enhancement. It remains hypointense on the venous and delayed phases of contrast enhancement. Which one of the following is the most likely diagnosis?
    a. Ductal adenocarcinoma
    b. Insulinoma
    c. Simple pancreatic cyst
    d. Gastrinoma
    e. Glucagonoma

39. A 45 year old female has a CT for abdominal pain and weight loss. Findings include a soft-tissue mass at the root of the small bowel mesentery with eccentric calcifications and tethering of adjacent small bowel loops resulting in a moderate degree of small bowel obstruction. There is a desmoplastic reaction within the surrounding mesentery. Which one of the following is the most likely diagnosis?
    a. Lymphoma
    b. Carcinoid tumour
    c. Melanoma metastases
    d. Tuberculosis
    e. Paraganglioma

40. A 50 year old female presents to A&E with acute abdominal pain. On examination there is point tenderness over an area in the right iliac fossa. CT reveals a well-defined triangular area of high-attenuation fat density anteriorly in the lower right abdomen. The large and small bowel are normal. Which one of the following is most likely?
    a. Segmental omental infarction
    b. Rectus haematoma
    c. Epiploic appendagitis
    d. Carcinoid tumour
    e. Mesenteric vein thrombosis

41. A 32 year old woman with no significant past medical history has a CT scan as an outpatient for right iliac fossa pain. No cause for the pain is discovered on this investigation. However, a 1 cm diameter, smoothly marginated, circular, homogenous area of tissue is seen next to the splenic hilum. This area of tissue is isodense compared to normal splenic parenchyma. What is this most likely to be?
    a. Splenosis
    b. Splenunculus
    c. Lymphoma
    d. Splenic hamartoma
    e. Wandering spleen

42. A 58 year old male with unexplained elevated alkaline phosphatase has an MRCP and the 'double-duct' sign is observed. Which one of the following diagnoses is most likely to cause this finding?
    a. Acute pancreatitis
    b. Annular pancreas

c. Pancreas divisum

d. Periampullary tumour

e. Duodenal perforation

43. A 42 year old woman undergoes a CT abdomen and pelvis for the investigation of right upper quadrant pain and deranged liver function tests. On early post-intravenous contrast images there is prominent enhancement of the central liver and weak enhancement of the peripheral liver. This pattern is reversed on delayed images. In addition there is hypertrophy of the caudate lobe. Which one of the following would most likely explain these findings?

    a. Acute hepatitis

    b. Cirrhosis

    c. Budd–Chiari syndrome

    d. Portal hypertension

    e. Fatty liver

44. A 61 year old man undergoes CT abdomen and pelvis for characterisation of a well-defined hyperechoic area seen on ultrasound in the perihilar region of the liver. On CT the area is of decreased attenuation but has no obvious mass effect. There is no abnormal enhancement with intravenous contrast administration. Which one of the following diagnoses is most likely?

    a. Focal nodular hyperplasia

    b. Focal fatty infiltration

    c. Hepatic cyst

    d. Liver haemangioma

    e. Fibrolamellar carcinoma

45. A 39 year old woman has an ultrasound scan for right upper quadrant pain and jaundice which reveals biliary ductal dilatation to the level of the common hepatic duct adjacent to a stone in the gallbladder neck. The gallbladder is thick-walled and tender. MRCP confirms these findings and excludes common duct stones. Which one of the following is the most likely diagnosis?

    a. Primary sclerosing cholangitis

    b. Mirizzi syndrome

    c. Caroli's disease

    d. Fascioliasis

    e. Acute cholecystitis

46. A 48 year old male presents with abdominal pain, nausea and weight loss. Contrast-enhanced CT of the abdomen and pelvis reveals a heterogeneous, well-defined fatty mass at the root of the small bowel mesentery. The mesenteric vessels are surrounded but not distorted by the mass, and the vessels are surrounded by an apparent low-attenuation halo. The small bowel and right colon are normal. Which is the most likely diagnosis?

    a. Tuberculosis

    b. Mesenteric lymphadenitis

    c. Mesenteric panniculitis

    d. Radiation enteritis

    e. Mesenteric lipoma

47. A 76 year old male on ITU has a CT abdomen and pelvis for the investigation of abdominal pain, pyrexia and diarrhoea. The CT reveals 12 mm diffuse large bowel wall thickening with intense mucosal enhancement and low attenuation of the submucosa involving the entire colon including the rectum, and a small volume of ascites. Which one of the following diagnoses is the most likely to explain the above findings?
    a. Crohn's colitis
    b. Pseudomembranous colitis
    c. Ischaemic colitis
    d. Yersinia
    e. Giardiasis

48. A 41 year old female has an MRI liver following a solitary 3 cm lesion in the right lobe of the liver. The lesion is isointense on T1-weighted and slightly hyperintense to liver parenchyma on T2-weighted imaging. There is immediate intense homogenous enhancement with gadolinium in the arterial phase, which becomes isointense on the venous phase. A central scar is hypointense on T1 and hyperintense on T2-weighted sequences. Which one of the following is the most likely diagnosis?
    a. Adenoma
    b. Cavernous haemangioma
    c. Fibrolamellar carcinoma
    d. Regenerative nodules
    e. Focal nodular hyperplasia

49. A 71 year old woman with no significant past medical history has an abdominal ultrasound as part of an investigation for right upper quadrant pain, anaemia and weight loss. Multiple, poorly defined, markedly echogenic lesions are seen throughout the liver. Biopsy reveals these to be metastases. Which one of the following is most likely to be the primary tumour?
    a. Adenocarcinoma of the colon
    b. Melanoma
    c. Invasive ductal carcinoma of the breast
    d. Gastric cancer
    e. Pancreatic ductal adenocarcinoma

50. A 51 year old male patient has a barium swallow for the investigation of dysphagia. This shows a 10 cm tapered stricture in the mid oesophagus along with multiple fine linear projections perpendicular to the lumen, each 3–4 mm long, in this segment. There are occasional tertiary contractions and mild gastro-oesophageal reflux. What is the most likely diagnosis?
    a. Chagas disease
    b. Oesophageal intramural pseudodiverticulosis
    c. Oesophageal varices
    d. Cytomegalovirus infection
    e. Oesophageal carcinoma

51. A 25 year old female becomes unwell six hours after induced delivery for pre-eclampsia with severe right upper quadrant pain, oedema and nausea. CT of the abdomen and pelvis reveals copious ascites and multiple wedge-shaped areas of liver non-enhancement

consistent with hepatic infarction. Which of the following is the most likely underlying cause?

a. Hepatic artery embolus
b. Portal vein thrombosis
c. SVC occlusion
d. HELLP syndrome
e. Splenic vein thrombosis

52. A 47 year old female with a history of surgery for breast carcinoma is referred for ultrasound after liver function tests show a mildly elevated alkaline phosphatase. The bile ducts are normal but a 3 cm hyperechoic liver lesion is seen in the right lobe. CT is recommended, which shows a focal mass with nodular hyperenhancement of the periphery on arterial phase imaging becoming isointense to the background liver on delayed phase scanning at five minutes. Which one of the following is the most likely diagnosis?

a. Fibrolamellar carcinoma
b. Adenoma
c. Cavernous haemangioma
d. Adenocarcinoma metastases
e. Focal nodular hyperplasia

53. A 33 year old female presents to A&E with right upper quadrant pain, hypotensive and tachycardic. CT abdomen and pelvis reveals an 11 cm diameter well-defined heterogenous mass within the right lobe of the liver, predominantly of low density but with three focal areas of higher attenuation (>90 HU) within it. There is layered high-attenuation fluid within the subhepatic and right subdiaphragmatic space tracking down to the pelvis. Which one of the following is the correct combination of recommendations?

a. Adenoma – recommend surgical referral
b. Adenoma – recommend correct coagulopathy and rescan if it deteriorates
c. Adenoma – recommend endovascular embolisation
d. Metastatic hepatocellular carcinoma – recommend gastroenterology referral
e. Trauma – needs CT thorax to clear other injuries

54. A 54 year old male has a liver MR for characterisation of a 3 cm low-attenuation lesion found on staging CT for rectal carcinoma. Which one of the following characteristics would be most worrying for a metastasis rather than a benign lesion?

a. Peripheral washout on delayed imaging
b. Intense arterial enhancement
c. Peripheral nodular enhancement
d. Presence of a pseudocapsule
e. Low signal intensity on T1-weighted imaging

55. A 63 year old male has a CT abdomen and pelvis for the investigation of change in bowel habit and weight loss. A sigmoid tumour is demonstrated and there is a solitary liver metastasis. Which one of the following observations on CT would render the patient ineligible for curative resection of the liver metastasis?

a. Presence of a single peripheral left lower lobe pulmonary metastasis
b. Presence of splenic metastasis

c. Direct extension of the liver metastasis into the right adrenal gland
d. Involvement of the caudate lobe
e. Peritoneal metastases

56. An ultrasound of the abdomen is performed on a 21 year old female presenting to A&E with acute right iliac fossa pain, pyrexia, tenderness and guarding. Which one of the following findings would suggest perforation of the appendix?
a. Appendix diameter of 8 mm
b. Appendix wall thickness of 4 mm
c. Decreased resistance of arterial waveform
d. Loss of visualisation of hyperechoic submucosa
e. Increased echogenicity of surrounding fat

57. A 52 year old male with a metal heart valve has a transrectal ultrasound performed to stage rectal carcinoma as MRI is contraindicated. A 3 cm hypoechoic mass is identified from three to seven o'clock in the lower rectum. It extends through an inner hypoechoic layer and into the outer hypoechoic layer, but the outermost hyperechoic layer is intact and unaffected. What is the correct T staging (TNM system) based on these observations?
a. T0
b. T1
c. T2
d. T3
e. T4

58. A 73 year old female has a CT abdomen and pelvis for the investigation of anaemia and weight loss. Massive splenomegaly (30 cm) is present with no other abnormalities. Which of the following conditions is most likely to be the underlying cause?
a. Sarcoidosis
b. Felty's syndrome
c. Chronic myeloid leukaemia
d. Haemochromatosis
e. Non-Hodgkin's lymphoma

59. A 57 year old diet-compliant male patient with coeliac disease has a CT abdomen and pelvis for the investigation of cachexia and two stone weight loss over six months. A 7 cm segment of ileum shows mild dilatation and circumferential thickening, with multiple low-attenuation mesenteric and para-aortic lymph nodes. Which one of the following is the most likely diagnosis?
a. Tuberculosis
b. Gastro-intestinal lymphoma
c. Coeliac disease
d. Whipple disease
e. Crohn's disease

60. A 60 year old male has an abdominal ultrasound for the investigation of deranged LFTs. A 2 cm hyperechoic mass is seen at the porta hepatis. There is dilatation of the right and left hepatic ducts but the common bile duct is of normal calibre. A PET-CT is

performed which shows an FDG-avid lesion corresponding to the abnormality on ultrasound and no other findings. Which of the following is the most likely diagnosis?
a. Caroli's disease
b. Klatskin tumour
c. Periampullary tumour
d. Primary sclerosing cholangitis
e. Biliary cystadenoma

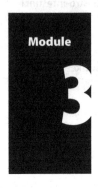

Gastro-intestinal – Answers

1. c. Hypoperistalsis in the upper third of the oesophagus
The oesophagus is the most commonly involved location of the gastro-intestinal tract in patients with scleroderma. Smooth muscle atrophy causes hypoperistalsis and eventually aperistalsis in the lower two-thirds of the oesophagus. The upper third of the oesophageal wall contains skeletal muscle and is therefore unaffected by the disease process.
(Ref: Dahnert p. 863)

2. d. Ipsilateral rib fractures
All are potential associated injuries and should be actively searched for in the context of blunt abdominal trauma. Rib fractures are found in up to 50% of patients with splenic injuries and as such are the most common association. The left kidney is injured in 10% of patients with splenic injury, and diaphragm rupture is even rarer. Diaphragm rupture may be difficult to appreciate on axial slices, and may be more evident on coronal reformats.
(Ref: Dahnert p. 807)

3. a. Type B
Congenital TE fistula and oesophageal atresia occur in approximately 1 in 4000 live births. They are divided into five subtypes, A to E. Type C is the most common, comprising 75% of all types and involves oesophageal atresia with a distal TE fistula. Type D involves oesopha-geal atresia with both proximal and distal TE fistula, and type E is a TE fistula without oesophageal atresia. Therefore types C to E do not typically present with gasless abdomen. Type B is oesophageal atresia with a proximal TE fistula; there is no communication between the trachea and the distal oesophagus, and therefore a gasless abdomen is typical. Type A is oesophageal atresia without TE fistula and therefore may also present with a gasless abdomen, but is not a listed option.
(Ref: Dahnert p. 817)

4. e. Presence of haustral markings
Sigmoid and caecal volvulus can sometimes be difficult to differentiate on plain abdominal film. With caecal volvulus the haustral markings are typically present, whereas these are usually absent in sigmoid volvulus. The pelvic overlap, liver overlap and coffee bean signs are typical of sigmoid volvulus. In sigmoid volvulus the apex lies high in the abdomen underneath the left hemi-diaphragm, typically above the level of T10.
(Ref: Grainger & Allison p. 597)

5. b. Epiploic appendagitis
Epiploic appendagitis is inflammation of one of the epiploic appendages of the colon, with the sigmoid being the commonest site. It typically presents with acute abdominal pain and

is an important radiological diagnosis as it can often mimic appendicitis, and management is conservative. The diagnosis is usually made on CT with the features described in the question. Ultrasound is rarely used for diagnosis, and features include a non-compressible hyperechoic mass with hypoechoic margins.
(Ref: Grainger & Allison p. 692, p. 722)

6. a. Typhlitis
Typhlitis, or neutropaenic enterocolitis, is acute inflammation of the caecum, ascending colon, terminal ileum or appendix. It is typically described in children with neutropaenia secondary to lymphoma, leukaemia and immunosuppression. Concentric, often marked, bowel wall thickening with pericolic inflammatory changes is typical, and such changes in a young immunosuppressed child should raise suspicion of typhlitis as a cause. Perforation is a risk factor and therefore contrast examinations are usually avoided.
(Ref: Brant & Helms p. 857)

7. d. Facial angiofibromas
MEN type 3 is a non-inherited syndrome primarily composing medullary thyroid carcinoma, phaeochromocytomas and mucosal neuromas of the gastro-intestinal tract. Other features include prognathism, marfanoid appearance and cutaneous neuromas. Facial angiofibromas are associated with MEN type 1 and occur in greater than 80% of cases.
(Refs: Dahnert p. 733; Grainger & Allison p. 1713)

8. b. Gastrinoma
Pancreatic adenocarcinoma is a hypovascular lesion. Macrocystic adenoma is also hypovascular, and is only rarely found in the head of the pancreas, with a predilection for the tail. The differential therefore lies between insulinoma and gastrinoma. Although both CT and MR imaging characteristics are similar, the majority of insulinomas are less than 1 cm in size, whereas gastrinomas tend to be larger at presentation with an average size of approximately 3 cm. Gastrinoma is associated with peptic ulceration and Zollinger–Ellison syndrome.
(Ref: Dahnert p. 735)

9. c. Carcinoid tumour
Of the options listed, carcinoid tumour is the only primary tumour that typically causes hypervascular liver metastases. Other causes of hypervascular liver metastases are pancreatic islet cell tumours, phaeochromocytoma and renal cell carcinoma. Stomach, breast, lung and colon cancers are associated with hypovascular liver metastases. Liver metastases from carcinoid tumours are more common with increasing size of the primary tumour. The incidence of metastases depends on the location of the primary tumour, where approximately 30% of carcinoids of the ileum metastasise compared to less than 5% of carcinoids of the appendix.
(Refs: Chapman & Nakielny 2003 p. 294; Dahnert p. 811)

10. a. Leiomyoma
Oesophageal leiomyoma is the most common benign submucosal tumour of the oesophagus, typically occurring in young men. The classical features of oesophageal leiomyoma include a smooth intramural mass in the lower or middle third of the oesophagus with

intact overlying mucosa. It is the only tumour of the oesophagus that calcifies, although calcification is rare.
(Ref: Grainger & Allison p. 615)

11. d. Hepatic artery invasion

The only widely recognised absolute contraindication to curative surgical resection of the options listed is invasion of the hepatic artery. Invasion of the splenic and portal veins are relative contraindications as long as the veins are not completely occluded. Invasion of the second part of the duodenum is not a contraindication as it is resected at surgery. Other features that make the tumour unsuitable for curative resection are distant metastases, ascites, distant organ invasion, SMA/coeliac/aortic invasion and involved lymph nodes outside the boundaries of the resection.
(Refs: Grainger & Allison p. 801; Saclarides *et al.* p. 293)

12. c. Schatzki ring

All are reasonable differentials for a mid-oesophageal stricture, albeit with varying degrees of frequency, with the exception of a Schatzki ring which is found in the lower oesophagus. It occurs near the squamocolumnar junction and is associated with reflux. It is non-distensible and best seen in the prone position on barium swallow examinations. Schatzki rings are often asymptomatic, but oesophageal dilatation may be required where dysphagia is severe.
(Refs: Chapman & Nakielny 2003 p. 229; Dahnert p. 867)

13. b. Cystadenocarcinoma of the appendix

The CT findings described are consistent with pseudomyxoma peritonei. This describes abdominal distension secondary to the accumulation of large quantities of gelatinous ascites. It is most commonly caused by cystadenocarcinoma of the appendix in males and cystadenocarcinoma of the ovary in females. Surgical debulking and intraperitoneal chemotherapy may be offered as a treatment. Bowel obstruction is a frequent complication that may necessitate surgery.
(Ref: Dahnert p. 866)

14. c. Ischaemic colitis

Crohn's colitis is relatively unlikely due to lack of prior history or small bowel involvement and age of the patient. Ulcerative colitis and pseudomembranous colitis are both unlikely as the rectum is usually involved in these two conditions. Infectious colitis does not normally affect the left-sided colon only, regardless of the underlying pathogen. Ischaemic colitis is the most likely diagnosis of those listed. It typically affects a segment of bowel, with the majority of cases having left-sided colonic involvement.
(Ref: Weissleder *et al.*)

15. c. Small bowel enteroclysis

Small bowel enteroclysis is the most appropriate examination. CT is sensitive for high-grade obstruction as it will readily identify the level of obstruction and can demonstrate complications such as ischaemia and perforation. Enteroclysis is the preferred investigation for recurrent low-grade obstruction as it is more likely to demonstrate the presence of a transition point (for example from non-obstructing adhesions) because the bowel is distended.

The examination involves passing a nasojejunal tube just distal to the duodenojejunal flexure and distending the small bowel using either dilute barium or a double-contrast examination with high-density barium and methylcellulose.
(Ref: Chapman & Nakielny 2001 p. 64)

16. e. Adenoma

The lesion is most likely to be a hepatic adenoma. None of the other diagnoses typically share these imaging characteristics. Adenomas are benign growths of hepatocytes and are most commonly seen in young women, particularly associated with oral contraceptive use. Eighty per cent are solitary and found in the right lobe of the liver. The high signal on T1-weighted sequences is due to the presence of fat and/or haemorrhage and can distinguish between this and many other lesions in the liver which tend to be of low T1 signal on MR (e.g. metastases, HCC, haemangiomas and FNH). Occasionally, imaging features can overlap with FNH and the two lesions can be difficult to distinguish. However, the majority of FNH lesions are less than 5 cm in size, whereas adenomas tend to be larger.
(Ref: Dahnert p. 719)

17. c. Fibrolamellar carcinoma

Fibrolamellar carcinoma occurs in young adults in the absence of normal risk factors for hepatocellular carcinoma. On ultrasound, fibrolamellar carcinoma is of mixed or increased echogenicity, and the hyperechoic central scar is often evident. On unenhanced CT the lesion is of low attenuation, displaying heterogenous enhancement with intravenous contrast administration. The central scar is typically of low signal on both T1- and T2-weighted imaging, which can help differentiate it from FNH (whose scar typically is of low signal on T1 but high signal on T2-weighted imaging). The central scar is present in up to 60% of patients. Calcifications are present in up to 55% and are more common than in hepatocellular carcinoma.
(Ref: Dahnert p. 726)

18. b. Intraductal papillary mucinous tumour of the pancreas

Intraductal papillary mucinous tumour (IPMT) of the pancreas is a rare tumour. It tends to present in the elderly population and can be a cause of recurrent pancreatitis. Two recognised types include main duct IPMT, in which the main pancreatic duct is dilated, and branch duct IPMT, in which the main duct is usually uninvolved. It is a risk factor for mucinous carcinoma of the pancreas. Pancreatic atrophy is often present. Imaging characteristics are often similar to those seen in chronic pancreatitis, although calcification is not a feature of IPMT.
(Ref: Dahnert p. 727)

19. a. Peutz–Jeghers

Peutz–Jeghers syndrome is most consistent with these findings. It is an autosomal dominant syndrome but often arises as a spontaneous mutation. Hamartomas are found throughout the gastro-intestinal tract, with the exception of the oesophagus. The polyps have almost no malignant potential, but life expectancy is decreased due to associated cancers arising in the stomach, duodenum, colon and ovary. Gardner's syndrome and familial polyposis are both associated with small bowel adenomas in approximately 5% of cases. Cowden's syndrome does involve hamartomatous polyps, but these are typically rectosigmoid, and small bowel involvement is not a feature. Small bowel polyps are not a feature of Turcot's syndrome. (Ref: Weissleder *et al.*)

20. d. Gardner's syndrome

Gardner's syndrome is an autosomal dominant condition with colonic polyps present in all patients. Small bowel, duodenal and stomach polyps are also a feature. Extra-intestinal features include osteomas of membranous bone (typically the mandible as described in the question), other soft-tissue tumours and periampullary carcinomas. Osteomas are not a feature of the other conditions. Cronkhite–Canada syndrome and Peutz–Jegher syndrome are associated with multiple hamartomatous polyps of the colon and stomach. Cronkhite–Canada syndrome is a sporadic non-familial disorder. Lynch syndrome, or hereditary non-polyposis colorectal carcinoma (HNPCC), is associated with increased risk of colorectal adenomas and other malignancies such as endometrial and other gastro-intestinal tract malignancies.
(Refs: Dahnert p. 833; Grainger & Allison p. 683)

21. e. T3N1M0

T1 tumour is disease confined to the pancreas and less than 2 cm in diameter. T2 tumour is also confined to the pancreas but greater than 2 cm in diameter. As the tumour extends beyond the boundary of the pancreas, it is at least T3. Invasion of the coeliac or superior mesenteric arteries would make this a T4 tumour, but as these features are not present it is T3. The presence of regional nodes make it N1 rather than N0 (no nodes involved), and there is no metastatic disease so it is M0. Therefore the correct radiological stage is T3N1M0.
(Ref: Kochman p. 389)

22. d. Adenomyomatosis of the gallbladder

The correct diagnosis is adenomyomatosis. This is an uncommon condition, more common in females, and is associated with gallstones in the majority of cases. It is characterised by generalised or focal mural thickening with intramural diverticula (Rokitansky–Aschoff sinuses). The ultrasound artefact from cholesterol crystals in the sinuses produces bright 'comet-tail' reverberation artefacts.
(Ref: Chapman & Nakielny 2003 p. 276)

23. a. Primary sclerosing cholangitis

These ultrasound and ERCP features are typical of primary sclerosing cholangitis, which is an idiopathic condition characterised by progressive fibrosis of the biliary tree. It primarily affects young men with inflammatory bowel disease (more common in ulcerative colitis than Crohn's) although pancreatitis, liver cirrhosis and chronic active hepatitis are other associated conditions. Primary biliary cirrhosis may also cause scattered areas of focal intrahepatic duct dilatation, but this condition is much more common in females and the extrahepatic ducts are not involved.
(Ref: Dahnert p. 699)

24. c. Choledochal cyst

The only one of the listed diagnoses that would have both these features on HIDA scan is a choledochal cyst. This is a congenital condition characterised by dilatation of the common

bile duct and common hepatic duct. Patients typically present in childhood with right upper quadrant pain, a mass and/or obstructive jaundice. Although the diagnosis is usually made with MRCP, HIDA scan can show typical features that include a photopaenic area in the liver representing the dilated CBD/CHD. Although a hepatic cyst would also show a photopaenic area within the liver, small bowel visualisation would be expected. Congenital biliary atresia would cause lack of small bowel visualisation, but the whole liver would take up HIDA and photopaenia would not be present.
(Ref: Dahnert p. 703)

25. c. Pneumoperitoneum
Whilst uncommon, the appearances seen on plain film are consistent with massive pneumo-peritoneum. The oval radiolucency is called the 'football sign' and arises due to free air collecting anterior to the intra-abdominal viscera. This sign is only seen in 2% of adults with pneumoperitoneum due to the large quantities of air required to produce it. It is much more common in infants who may present at a later stage. The opacity in the right upper quadrant is produced by air outlining the falciform ligament, which again is a sign of pneumoperitoneum. Causes of perforation in this age group include trauma, intussusception and complications of Meckel's diverticulum.
(Ref: Rampton J. The football sign. *Radiology* 2004; **231**: 81–82)

26. b. Menetrier's disease
Menetrier's disease is a condition characterised by gastric mucosal hypertrophy and protein-losing enteropathy. It is often associated with anaemia. The changes are most marked along the greater curve and the antrum is spared in approximately 50% of cases. Gastric lymphoma typically involves the antrum. With gastric adenocarcinoma and linitis plastica, stomach distension is not typically preserved.
(Ref: Grainger & Allison p. 637)

27. c. Coeliac disease
Jejunal dilatation and jejunisation of the ileal loops are characteristic features of coeliac disease. This is an immunological intolerance to gluten that causes villous atrophy in the small intestine. In Whipple disease there is thickening of the jejunal and duodenal mucosal folds but typically no luminal dilatation. Dilatation of the small bowel does occur with lymphoma but jejunisation of the ileum is not a feature.
(Ref: Chapman & Nakielny 2003 p. 247)

28. a. Hydatid cyst
The most likely diagnosis is hydatid cyst disease. This condition is caused by infection of the liver with the parasite *Echinococcus granulosus*. Blood eosinophilia is present in up to 50% of patients. It is more common in the right lobe of the liver and is multiple in 20% of cases. Daughter cysts are typical. Percutaneous aspiration of the cyst is positive for hydatid disease in 70%.
(Ref: Dahnert p. 711)

29. c. Gallstone ileus
Specific signs of gallstone ileus can be seen on the plain abdominal film in up to 40% of patients. Fifty per cent of patients have evidence of small bowel obstruction and up to 30%

have gas in the biliary tree. Biliary tree gas is typically more prominent centrally and spares the periphery of the liver, whereas portal venous gas is more easily visualised in the periphery of the liver, which may be associated with small bowel infarction. The gallstone most frequently lodges in the terminal ileum, but is often not seen on the plain film. The presence of small bowel obstruction, pneumobilia and a visible stone are called Rigler's triad.
(Refs: Dahnert p. 832; Grainger & Allison p. 595)

30. b. Plain abdominal film
Toxic megacolon is a complication of ulcerative colitis, Crohn's and other forms of acute colitis. It has a poor prognosis with up to 20% mortality. Plain abdominal radiography should be the first line investigation for suspected toxic megacolon, and can be repeated 24 or 48 hourly if necessary. It can often confirm the diagnosis without the need for CT, which is especially useful when considering radiation dose issues in this group of young patients. Typical features on plain film include transverse colon dilatation >5.5 cm, loss of normal haustral folds, thumbprinting of the colon and the presence of mucosal islands (pseudopolyps). CT better demonstrates potential complications of toxic megacolon such as perforation of the bowel.
(Ref: Grainger & Allison p. 696)

31. a. Crohn's disease
These features are highly suggestive of Crohn's disease. Signs on double contrast barium enema that favour a diagnosis of Crohn's disease over ulcerative colitis include apthoid ulcers, deep ulcers, discontinuous ulceration, rectal sparing, pseudodiverticulae, fistulae and abscess formation. Ulcerative colitis can be suggested by rectal involvement, continuous pathology with no skip lesions and the presence of mucosal granularity. However, these features may also be present in Crohn's and are not specific for ulcerative colitis. Although tuberculosis is a mimic, colonic involvement in this pattern is uncommon compared with Crohn's disease.
(Ref: Dahnert p. 818)

32. e. Giardiasis
All the stems are potential causes for these symptoms in a patient with AIDS, however giardiasis is the most likely cause given these imaging appearances. *Cytomegalovirus* most typically affects the caecum, and tuberculosis affects the caecum and ileocaecal valve. *Mycobacterium avium intracellulare* can affect the ileum and jejunum but does not usually cause spasm. *Cryptosporidium* affects the duodenum and the jejunum can be affected, but dilatation is more common than spasm.
(Ref: Weissleder *et al.*)

33. a. Angiodysplasia
The typical angiographic feature of a Meckel's diverticulum is presence of the vitelline artery. Meckel's diverticulum also typically (although not exclusively) presents in younger patients. With diverticulosis, radiation enteritis and polyps, one might expect an abnormal barium enema, and in addition these angiographic features are not typical. Angiodysplasia is the second most common cause of gastro-intestinal bleed in the elderly population after diverticular disease. It is due to dilatation of the submucosal vessels and occurs most

commonly on the right side of the colon. Angiographic features include visualisation of a cluster of vessels on the antimesenteric border, early filling of the ileocolic vein in the arterial phase and delayed emptying of the same vein.
(Ref: Dahnert p. 802)

34. e. Tailgut cyst

Tailgut cysts or cystic hamartomas are presacral, multilocular, mucous-secreting cysts found distal to the normal embryonic termination of the hindgut. Small cysts may be asymptomatic, but larger cysts may present with rectal pain or bleeding, constipation, anal fistulae or recurrent rectal abscesses. A long and tail-like coccyx is often associated, and can help distinguish between many other cystic lesions in this region. Malignant transformation is a complication, most commonly adenocarcinoma. Duplication cysts are most often unilocular unless complicated by haemorrhage or infection, a meningocele is likely to arise from the sacral foramina, piercing the presacral fascia, and dermoid tumour would be expected to contain fat or layering of contents as seen in dermoid tumours in other locations.
(Ref: Stevenson & Hall p. 782)

35. a. Coeliac disease

All of these may cause malabsorption. Amyloid can cause dilatation but also causes diffuse thickening of the valvulae conniventes throughout the small bowel. With Whipple disease and eosinophilic gastroenteritis, one would not see dilatation of the bowel, but thickening of the mucosa is again a prominent feature. Giardiasis causes thickening and marked distortion of the mucosal folds in the duodenum and jejunum. One of the hallmark features of untreated coeliac disease is jejunal dilatation. Typically the mucosal folds are of normal thickness.
(Ref: Weissleder *et al.*)

36. a. Pyloric muscle wall thickness of 2 mm

Hypertrophic pyloric stenosis presents between four and six weeks of life with non-bilious vomiting, typically in first-born males. A palpable olive-shaped mass is a sign with reported sensitivity of up to 80%, but ultrasound is the most frequently used imaging modality. Typical ultrasound features include the target sign (central hyperechoic mucosa with surrounding hypoechoic pyloric muscle), the nipple sign (pyloric mucosa indenting the gastric antrum), pyloric canal length >16 mm, transverse pyloric diameter >13 mm and pyloric muscle wall thickness >3 mm. Pyloric stenosis can be difficult to differentiate radiologically from infantile pylorospasm. Typically with pylorospasm the appearances change with time, and so if the pyloric muscle thickness is measured at less than 3 mm this makes infantile pylorospasm the more likely diagnosis.
(Ref: Dahnert p. 842)

37. b. Amiodarone use

The normal liver is between 30 and 70 HU on unenhanced CT, and should be 10–15 HU lower than spleen density. On portal venous phase the liver will be approximately 25 HU less than the spleen. Amiodarone contains iodine and can cause the liver to appear of increased density on CT. Other causes include cisplatin use, haemochromatosis, Wilson disease and glycogen storage diseases. The more common finding on CT is a liver of

decreased density due to a fatty liver. This has many causes including alcohol use, steroids, chemotherapy, diabetes and nutritional causes.
(Ref: Weissleder *et al.*)

38. a. Ductal adenocarcinoma
Insulinoma tends to be hyperintense on contrast-enhanced images. Gastrinoma is usually hyperintense on STIR imaging and on contrast-enhanced sequences. In a series of 25 patients, an article by Chandarana *et al.* showed that pancreatic adenocarcinomas were either iso- or hypointense on T1-weighted imaging and iso- or hyperintense on T2 or STIR. All adenocarcinomas were hypointense to pancreatic parenchyma during the arterial phase of gadolinium enhancement on MR, 80% remained hypointense in the venous phase of enhancement and 68% remained hypointense in the delayed phase.
(Ref: Chandarana H *et al.* Signal characteristic and enhancement patterns of pancreatic adenocarcinoma: evaluation with dynamic gadolinium enhanced MRI. *Clinical Radiology* 2007; **62**: 876–883)

39. b. Carcinoid tumour
These features are typical of carcinoid tumour. The desmoplastic reaction appears on CT as thickened mesentery in a radiating pattern away from the soft-tissue mass, with beading of the mesenteric vascular bundles.
(Ref: Hyland R & Chalmers A. CT features of jejunal pathology. *Clinical Radiology* 2007; **62**: 1154–1162)

40. a. Segmental omental infarction
Segmental omental infarction is the most likely cause and most commonly affects the right half of the greater omentum. It mimics surgical pathology such as appendicitis. High-attenuation streaks in the omental fat with apparent 'mass effect' in the absence of any other findings is suggestive of the diagnosis. Point tenderness over the specific area of CT abnormality is often discovered. Management is conservative.
(Ref: Puylaert JB. Right-sided segmental infarction of the omentum: clinical, US and CT findings. *Radiology* 1992; **185**: 169–172)

41. b. Splenunculus
Splenunculus is most likely, and is often seen incidentally. It is much more common than splenosis and is more likely to occur at the splenic hilum than splenosis. A splenunculus, or accessory spleen, is present in up to 30% of people and is most often located near the splenic hilum, but can occur anywhere in the abdomen. Splenogonadal fusion is a recognised entity whereby the accessory splenic tissue is attached to the left ovary or testis. Splenosis occurs following trauma, whereby splenic tissue autotransplants elsewhere in the abdomen, and can also implant above the diaphragm if associated with diaphragm rupture. A wandering spleen denotes abnormal mobility of the spleen on long peritoneal ligaments.
(Refs: Dahnert p. 692; Grainger & Allison p. 1768)

42. d. Periampullary tumour
The 'double-duct' sign is dilatation of the main pancreatic duct and the common bile duct as seen at ERCP and MRCP, and less commonly with CT and ultrasound. It occurs due to an obstructing lesion at the ampulla, most commonly a carcinoma of the head of the pancreas

(in up to 77% of cases) or a carcinoma of the ampulla of Vater (in up to 52% of cases). The sign may be absent if there is an accessory pancreatic duct or when the main pancreatic duct drains into the minor papilla.
(Ref: Ahualli J. The double duct sign. *Radiology* 2007; **244**: 314–315)

43. c. Budd–Chiari syndrome
Budd–Chiari syndrome is outflow obstruction of the hepatic veins due to a wide variety of causes, but two-thirds are idiopathic. CT features include 'flip-flop' enhancement pattern as described in the question, ascites, hepatosplenomegaly, gallbladder wall thickening and increased portal vein diameter. An enlarged caudate lobe is seen in up to 88%, which enhances normally due its venous drainage passing directly into the IVC.
(Ref: Dahnert p. 694)

44. b. Focal fatty infiltration
Focal fatty infiltration occurs typically in the periportal and centrilobar regions of the liver and is commonest adjacent to the falciform ligament. Ultrasound features include a hyperechoic area with geographic margins. CT shows an area of decreased attenuation which does not alter the course of blood vessels or liver contour. The lesions are of high signal on T1-weighted MR imaging, and isointense or low signal on T2-weighted imaging. Haemangiomas would also typically be of increased echogenicity on ultrasound, but would be expected to show increased peripheral enhancement with intravenous contrast on CT.
(Refs: Chapman & Nakielny 2003 p. 292; Dahnert p. 713)

45. b. Mirizzi syndrome
Mirizzi syndrome is narrowing of the common hepatic duct caused by a gallstone impacted in the neck of the gallbladder or the cystic duct. The stricture is smooth and often concave to the right as seen on ERCP. Fistulae can develop between the gallbladder and the common duct, and the stone may pass into the common duct. It is associated with acute cholecystitis. Fascioliasis is caused by liver fluke infestation which may cause bile duct wall thickening and multiple hepatic abscesses. Caroli's disease is a congenital disorder characterised by cystic dilatation of the intrahepatic bile ducts.
(Ref: Grainger & Allison p. 778)

46. c. Mesenteric panniculitis
These CT findings are typical of mesenteric panniculitis. This is an idiopathic, indolent condition characterised by inflammation of the small bowel mesentery adipose tissue. Fibrosis can predominate, in which case the CT appearances are of an infiltrative soft-tissue mass with soft-tissue density strands radiating away from it. In this situation it has similar appearance to lymphoma, carcinoid or desmoid tumours or retroperitoneal fibrosis, and biopsy is required to differentiate. Mesenteric panniculitis often presents with non-specific symptoms such as abdominal pain, weight loss, nausea, vomiting and pyrexia, and is usually indolent and self-limiting.
(Ref: Grainger & Allison p. 717)

47. b. Pseudomembranous colitis
Pseudomembranous colitis results from overgrowth of *Clostridium difficile* most commonly due to broad spectrum antibiotic use in the hospital population. Ascites is often present in severe

cases and wall thickening >10 mm is highly suggestive of this diagnosis. A layered pattern of enhancement is often present in severe cases with oedema in the submucosa producing low attenuation in the wall, deep to the enhancing mucosa. The accordion sign is caused by marked submucosal oedema producing thickening of the colonic haustra. The rectum is involved in the majority of cases but any location within the large bowel may be involved. (Ref: Dahnert p. 865)

48. e. Focal nodular hyperplasia
These imaging features are typical of focal nodular hyperplasia. This is the second most common benign liver tumour and typically occurs in women more often than in men. Adenomas are usually larger, enhance less brightly and do not typically have a central fibrous scar. Cavernous haemangiomas are usually high signal on T2-weighted images, and of blood pool intensity on contrast-enhanced T1-weighted images. Fibrolamellar carcinoma also has a central scar, but this is typically of low signal intensity on T2-weighted imaging. Regenerative nodules show high signal intensity on unenhanced T1-weighted imaging and do not have a scar. (Ref: Marin D *et al.* Focal nodular hyperplasia: typical and atypical MRI findings with emphasis on the use of contrast media. *Clinical Radiology* 2008; **63**: 577–585)

49. a. Adenocarcinoma of the colon
The most common primary tumours that cause brightly echogenic liver metastases are colonic adenocarcinoma, treated breast cancer and hepatoma. The differential here therefore lies between breast cancer and colon cancer. Colon cancer makes up at least 50% of highly echogenic metastases. In addition the question states that the patient has no significant past medical history, and therefore treated breast cancer is unlikely. (Refs: Chapman & Nakielny 2003 p. 288; Dahnert p. 731)

50. b. Oesophageal intramural pseudodiverticulosis
Oesophageal intramural diverticulosis relates to dilated excretory ducts of the deep mucous glands of the oesophagus. They are best demonstrated on barium swallow and have the classical appearance as described in the question. The pseudodiverticular can appear to float outside the oesophagus when no communication with the lumen is seen. Most patients have dysphagia at presentation and associated conditions include diabetes, candida infection, oesophagitis, stricture and alcohol abuse. (Ref: Dahnert p. 828)

51. d. HELLP syndrome
Hepatic infarction is rare because of the dual blood supply to the liver via the hepatic arterial system and the portal venous system. Isolated pathology in either of these vascular supplies is unlikely to cause hepatic necrosis as the other supply will usually compensate. HELLP is characterised by haemolysis, elevated liver enzymes and low platelets and is one of the causes of liver infarction. (Ref: Dahnert p. 1045)

52. c. Cavernous haemangioma
Metastases may show peripheral enhancement with complete fill-in on delayed images, but they typically show complete rather than nodular peripheral enhancement and washout on delayed phase imaging. Only haemangiomas typically show peripheral nodular

enhancement. Cavernous haemangiomas are the most common benign liver tumours and are usually less than 4 cm in size. Seventy per cent are hyperechoic on ultrasound and they may show acoustic enhancement.
(Ref: Dahnert p. 721)

53. c. Adenoma – recommend endovascular embolisation

Adenomas are vascular lesions comprising hepatocytes. They may occasionally present with massive haemorrhage, and are the most common liver lesion to do so in young people. In this scenario there is active extravasation of contrast implying active bleeding and haemo-peritoneum. Urgent embolisation is the most appropriate treatment to halt bleeding. Conservative or surgical management is unlikely to provide rapid haemostasis. As a proportion of adenomas become malignant, they are usually removed surgically.
(Ref: Lee p. 854)

54. a. Peripheral washout on delayed imaging

Peripheral washout of contrast on delayed imaging is virtually diagnostic of malignancy. On post-gadolinium-enhanced T1-weighted images most metastases are hypovascular com-pared with the surrounding liver and are most conspicuous at the portal phase of enhance-ment. However, virtually all metastases exhibit a complete ring of peripheral enhancement, which is best seen in the early arterial phase.
(Ref: Mahfouz AE *et al.* Peripheral washout: a sign of malignancy on dynamic gadolinium-enhanced MR images of focal liver lesions. *Radiology* 1994; **190**: 49–52)

55. e. Peritoneal metastases

Generally accepted contraindications to liver resection would include uncontrollable extra-hepatic disease such as: non-treatable primary tumour; widespread pulmonary disease; locoregional recurrence; peritoneal disease; extensive nodal disease, such as retroperitoneal, mediastinal or portal nodes; and bone or CNS metastases. Patients with extrahepatic disease that should be considered for liver resection include: resectable/ablatable pulmonary metas-tases; resectable/ablatable isolated extrahepatic sites – for example, spleen, adrenal or resectable local recurrence; and local direct extension of liver metastases to, for example, the diaphragm or adrenal glands, which can be resected.
(Ref: Garden OJ *et al.* Guidelines for resection of colorectal cancer liver metastases. *Gut* 2006; **55**(Suppl III): iii1–iii8)

56. d. Loss of visualisation of hyperechoic submucosa

The use of ultrasound for the diagnosis of acute appendicitis is particularly useful in children and women of child-bearing age. Findings indicating acute appendicitis include a tubular non-compressible blind-ending structure with diameter >6 mm and wall thickness >2 mm, although these signs do not necessarily indicate perforation. Features suggesting perforation include a fluid collection adjacent to the appendix, gas bubbles near the appendix and loss of visualisation of the submucosal layer.
(Ref: Dahnert p. 803)

57. c. T2

The layers of the rectum are well demonstrated at transrectal ultrasound. The innermost hyperechoic layer represents the balloon-mucosa interface, the middle hyperechoic layer

represents the submucosa and the outermost hyperechoic layer represents the serosa. The tumour described in the question extends through the submucosa into the muscularis propria (outer hypoechoic layer) but does not involve the serosa. T1 disease is limited to the submucosa, T2 is limited to the muscularis propria, T3 extends through the serosa and T4 represents invasion of adjacent organs. The correct staging for the tumour described in the question is therefore T2.
(Ref: Grainger & Allison p. 815)

58. c. Chronic myeloid leukaemia
Splenomegaly is a relatively common finding in many different diseases, but massive splenomegaly always indicates underlying pathology. Although there is no unifying defin-ition, it is often recognised to be enlargement of the spleen into the left lower quadrant of the abdomen or crossing the midline. All the options listed are causes of splenomegaly, however chronic myeloid leukaemia is the only listed cause of massive splenomegaly. Other causes of massive splenomegaly include Gaucher's disease, malaria, myelofibrosis, schisto-somiasis and Leishmaniasis.
(Ref: Doherty & Way p. 633)

59. b. Gastro-intestinal lymphoma
Hypoattenuating lymph nodes can be attributed to many causes, but lymphoma and tuberculosis are the most common. Lymphoma of the gastro-intestinal tract most com-monly affects the ileum, although lymphoma associated with coeliac disease most com-monly affects the jejunum. Although 90% of tuberculosis of the gastro-intestinal tract occurs in the ileum, lymphoma is most likely in this scenario. Dilatation of the small bowel with lymphoma is common but obstruction is rare due to the soft pliable nature of the tumour.
(Ref: Dahnert p. 851)

60. b. Klatskin tumour
Klatskin tumours are the most common form of cholangiocarcinoma, representing tumour at the confluence of the hepatic ducts. The finding of a hyperechoic central porta hepatis mass at ultrasound is typical. Risk factors include inflammatory bowel disease, primary sclerosing cholangitis, Caroli's disease and cholecystolithiasis. Cholangiocarcinomas have a very poor prognosis with a five-year survival of less than 2%. They are FDG-avid and PET-CT is typically performed in the pre-operative evaluation of these tumours.
(Ref: Dahnert p. 696)

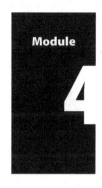
Genito-urinary, adrenal, obstetrics & gynaecology and breast – Questions

1. A 40 year old mother of three presents with menorrhagia and dysmenorrhoea. Transvaginal ultrasound shows an enlarged uterus with focal heterogeneous myometrial echotexture. The endometrium appears widened. T2-weighted MR imaging demonstrates focal widening of the junctional zone. There is a hypointense elongated myometrial mass with ill-defined margins. The mass contains foci of high signal on both T1- and T2-weighted imaging. The mass demonstrates contrast enhancement but to a lesser degree than the surrounding myometrium. What is the most likely diagnosis?
   a. Leiomyoma
   b. Endometrial carcinoma
   c. Adenomyosis
   d. Fibroma
   e. Haematoma

2. A 42 year old woman presents with post-coital bleeding. Transvaginal ultrasound shows the cervix to be enlarged, irregular and hypoechoic. MRI demonstrates a large cervical cancer with involvement of multiple pelvic lymph nodes. The left kidney is hydronephrotic. What is the most appropriate staging based on these findings?
   a. T1
   b. T2b
   c. T3a
   d. T3b
   e. T4

3. A 50 year old woman presents with pelvic pain and abdominal fullness. Ultrasound reveals ascites and a large hypoechoic ovarian mass with posterior acoustic enhancement. CT demonstrates a well-defined solid pelvic mass which shows poor contrast enhancement. There is also a right-sided pleural effusion. Follow-up imaging post-surgical resection shows no residual tumour and resolution of ascites. What is the most likely diagnosis?
   a. Serous cystadenocarcinoma
   b. Mucinous cystadenocarcinoma
   c. Ovarian fibroma
   d. Brenner tumour
   e. Massive ovarian oedema

4. A 34 year old man presents with a dull ache and a focal non-tender lesion in the right inguinal region. It is heterogeneous on ultrasound and CT. On MR, it has

a heterogeneous signal intensity on T1- and T2-weighted imaging, which enhances post-gadolinium. Which of the following is the likely diagnosis?
a. Haematoma
b. Lipoma of the cord
c. Neurofibroma
d. Abscess
e. Malignancy in an undescended testis

5. A 65 year old man undergoes a penile MR for staging of penile cancer. Which of the following is true?
a. Corpus spongiosum has a high signal on T1-weighted images
b. On T2-weighted images, the periurethral tissue has high signal intensity relative to the corpus spongiosum
c. Corpus spongiosum enhances more rapidly following gadolinium as compared to the corpora cavernosa
d. MR can reliably differentiate between Buck's fascia and tunica albuginea
e. A pelvic coil is preferred for local staging of penile cancers

6. A 69 year old man undergoes an MR for staging of prostate cancer. Which of the following is true regarding MR imaging of the prostate gland?
a. The zonal anatomy is best depicted on T1-weighted images
b. The central zone has a higher signal than the peripheral zone on T2-weighted images
c. The low signal intensity posterolateral to the capsule on T2-weighted imaging represents the seminal vesicles
d. The proximal urethra is usually identified easily
e. Post-contrast, the peripheral zone enhances more than the central zone

7. A 23 year old female has a renal ultrasound scan for recurrent urinary tract infections. The only abnormality detected is a 3 cm hyperechoic mass in the upper pole of the left kidney. She subsequently undergoes CT which shows the lesion to have an average HU of –10. Which of the following is the most likely diagnosis?
a. Renal cell carcinoma
b. Transitional cell carcinoma
c. Renal lymphoma
d. Angiomyolipoma
e. Renal abscess

8. An 84 year old diabetic female is investigated for recurrent *E. coli* urinary tract infections and microscopic haematuria. An intravenous urogram is performed, which shows numerous small filling defects in the ureter and small mural plaque-like defects within the bladder. Which one of the following is the most likely diagnosis?
a. Malakoplakia
b. Leukoplakia
c. Emphysematous cystitis
d. Emphysematous pyelonephritis
e. Pyeloureteritis cystica

9. A 65 year old male has a renal ultrasound scan for right flank pain which demonstrates a 7 cm solid mass within the right kidney with a hypoechoic centre. Subsequent CT scan of the chest, abdomen and pelvis reveals the lesion to have a low-attenuation central scar. There is no renal vein invasion or evidence of malignancy elsewhere in the body. Which of the following is the most likely diagnosis?
   a. Lymphoma of the kidney
   b. Transitional cell carcinoma
   c. Collecting duct tumour
   d. Oncocytoma
   e. Nephroblastoma

10. A 62 year old woman presents with two small masses in her right breast. These are well circumscribed masses in the upper outer quadrant. They show no calcification, no desmoplastic reaction and are not spiculated. They are thought to represent metastases to the breast. The most likely primary in a woman of this age is:
   a. Ovarian carcinoma
   b. Renal carcinoma
   c. Lymphoma
   d. Melanoma
   e. Bronchial carcinoma

11. A 24 year old woman attends A&E with lower abdominal pain and vaginal bleeding. A pregnancy test is positive. She is haemodynamically stable and an ultrasound is requested to confirm the presumed diagnosis of an ectopic pregnancy. Which of the following is the most common location for an ectopic pregnancy?
   a. Cervix
   b. Ovary
   c. Abdominal cavity
   d. Ampullary portion of the fallopian tube
   e. Interstitial portion of the fallopian tube

12. A 26 year old pregnant woman attends for an obstetric ultrasound at 37 weeks. She is shown to have polyhydramnios. Which of the following would be a possible cause?
   a. Cystic adenoid malformation
   b. Ventricular septal defect
   c. Infantile polycystic kidney disease
   d. Posterior urethral valves
   e. Intrauterine growth retardation

13. A 28 year old woman presents with a dull ache in her pelvis. Ultrasound shows a 7 cm well-defined ovarian cyst. A distinct echogenic nodule which causes dense acoustic shadowing is seen projecting into the cyst's lumen. What is the most likely diagnosis?
   a. Mature cystic teratoma
   b. Tubo-ovarian abscess
   c. Endometrioma
   d. Ovarian carcinoma
   e. Corpus luteum cyst

14. A 23 year old woman undergoes investigation for dyspareunia. Pelvic ultrasound was unremarkable. MRI demonstrates a 1 cm thin-walled ovoid cystic lesion at the anterolateral aspect of the upper vagina. It is homogeneously hypointense on T1 and shows marked hyperintensity on T2. What is the most likely diagnosis?
    a. Bartholin cyst
    b. Nabothian cyst
    c. Cervical fibroid
    d. Gartner duct cyst
    e. Cervical polyp

15. A 48 year old woman undergoes investigation for postmenopausal bleeding. Ultrasound shows a hyperechoic endometrial mass which contains several small cystic spaces. Power Doppler reveals a vessel at its base. On T2-weighted MR imaging the mass contains a central fibrous core with low signal intensity and small, well-delineated cysts showing marked high signal intensity. The central core enhances post-contrast administration. The junctional zone is intact. What is the most likely diagnosis?
    a. Endometrial hyperplasia
    b. Submucosal leiomyoma
    c. Submucosal fibroid
    d. Adenomyoma
    e. Endometrial polyp

16. A 36 year old man suffers pelvic fracture following a road traffic accident. On examination, blood is noted at the urethral meatus and the patient has urinary retention. Regarding urothelial injuries:
    a. Associated bladder injuries are seen in 50% of patients
    b. Anterior urethral injuries are commoner with pelvic fractures
    c. They are more commonly associated with pelvic fractures in females rather than males
    d. Posterior urethral injuries can be seen in up to 20% of pelvic fractures in males
    e. Impotence is a rare complication of male urethral injury

17. A 70 year old man undergoes an MR examination of the prostate to assess the stage of prostatic carcinoma. Which of the following is the least accurate?
    a. Obliteration of the rectoprostatic angle is suggestive of extracapsular spread
    b. Bladder and rectal involvement are best seen on coronal images
    c. Focal low signal in the seminal vesicles on T2-weighted imaging is a feature of invasion
    d. On T2-weighted images, prostate cancer usually demonstrates low signal intensity in contrast to the normal peripheral zone
    e. Prostatic volume measurements are bigger on CT than MR

18. A 28 year old woman suffers blunt injury to her abdomen following a road traffic accident. A polytrauma CT scan does not demonstrate any intra-abdominal injuries, but there are features indicating retroperitoneal injuries. Regarding these features, which of the following is true?
    a. Retroperitoneal air may indicate pulmonary injuries
    b. Haematomas in the posterior pararenal space do not extend into the pelvis

c. The most common region demonstrating retroperitoneal haemorrhage following trauma is usually around the aorto-caval region in the midline

d. Adrenal injuries are more common on the left

e. Low-attenuation fluid (<–20 HU) in the retroperitoneum is always indicative of injury to the pelvi-calyceal system or the ureters

19. A 45 year old male is diagnosed with renal cell carcinoma and is being worked up for curative nephrectomy. Which one of the following imaging modalities would you advise as being the most accurate at ruling out malignant renal vein invasion?
    a. Doppler ultrasound
    b. B-mode ultrasound
    c. CT
    d. MRI
    e. PET-CT

20. A 31 year old male is involved in a road traffic accident. The patient was catheterised immediately in A&E and the bladder was found to be empty. A trauma series CT is requested and a left-sided pelvic fracture is noted. A CT cystogram is therefore performed and bladder rupture is diagnosed. Which of the following signs would be an unexpected finding with this history?
    a. Contrast extravasation into the paracolic gutters
    b. Contrast extravasation into the perivesical fat
    c. Contrast extravasation into the anterior abdominal wall
    d. Flame-shaped contrast extravasation
    e. Contrast extravasation into the upper thigh

21. A 71 year old male undergoes renal CT for characterisation of a cystic renal mass. Which one of the following five features would classify the lesion as a Bosniak III lesion?
    a. Lack of enhancement
    b. Septation
    c. Minimally irregular wall
    d. Curvilinear calcification
    e. Uniform wall thickening

22. A 29 year old woman with a history of three previous failed pregnancies attends the ultrasound department for a scan. She has had a positive pregnancy test. Which of the following is not necessarily indicative of a failed pregnancy?
    a. A crown rump length of 11 mm with no heartbeat detectable on TA scan
    b. A crown rump length of 5 mm with no heartbeat detectable on TV scan
    c. A gestation sac, mean sac diameter >20 mm with no visible yolk sac
    d. A gestation sac, mean sac diameter >25 mm with no visible embryo
    e. A flat M mode scan

23. A 62 year old woman with Paget's disease of the nipple is also found to have a 2 cm spiculate mass in the subarealor region of her right breast suspicious for malignancy. The cancer most commonly associated with Paget's disease of the nipple is:
    a. Invasive ductal carcinoma
    b. Invasive lobular carcinoma

    c. Tubular carcinoma

    d. Ductal carcinoma in situ

    e. Medullary carcinoma

24. In a 72 year old man undergoing abdominal CT for ongoing lower abdominal pain, a 2 cm right-sided adrenal lesion is detected. He has no history of malignant disease. Which of the following parameters would be more in keeping with a malignant than a benign adrenal lesion?

    a. Size of 2.5 cm

    b. Hounsfield units of 8 on non-enhanced CT

    c. Washout of >60% when comparing non-enhanced CT with contrast-enhanced CT

    d. Loss of signal within the lesion on out-of-phase MRI imaging

    e. Maximum standardised uptake value >4 on FDG-PET

25. A 19 year old female presents with vague lower abdominal pain. Ultrasound shows a right 5 cm thin-walled unilocular ovarian cyst. Follow-up ultrasound six weeks later shows cyst regression. What is the most likely diagnosis?

    a. Corpus luteum cyst

    b. Endometrioma

    c. Serous cystadenoma

    d. Surface epithelial inclusion cyst

    e. Follicular cyst

26. A 14 year old girl presents with acute onset of right lower abdominal pain. She reports that she has had similar symptoms previously. Ultrasound shows an ovoid-shaped enlarged right-sided ovary containing multiple enlarged follicles. The ovarian stroma is echogenic compared to adjacent myometrium. There is peripheral blood flow on power Doppler and free fluid within the pelvis. What is the most likely diagnosis?

    a. Ovarian hyperstimulation

    b. Ovarian torsion

    c. Polycystic ovary syndrome

    d. Theca lutein cysts

    e. Serous cystadenoma

27. A female patient undergoes investigation for dysmenorrhea. She is obese, hirsute and has elevated luteinising hormone levels. Which of the following ultrasonographic findings is consistent with a diagnosis of polycystic ovarian syndrome?

    a. Ovarian volume >10 ml when no follicles measuring over 5 mm in diameter are present

    b. Ten or more follicles (3–12 mm diameter) present in an ovary

    c. Ovarian volume >15 ml when no follicles measuring over 10 mm in diameter are present

    d. Twelve or more follicles (3 mm diameter) present in an ovary

    e. Ovarian volume >10 ml when no follicles measuring over 10 mm in diameter are present

28. A 60 year old female presents with a large abdominal mass. CT demonstrates a large retroperitoneal fat-containing mass. Which of the following is true about the different fat-containing retroperitoneal masses?

   a. Predominantly low signal on T1-weighted and a high signal on T2-weighted images preclude a diagnosis of liposarcoma
   b. Calcification within a liposarcoma is usually associated with a better prognosis
   c. Lipomas are rare in the retroperitoneum
   d. An extremely FDG-avid retroperitoneal fat-containing tumour is almost certainly a liposarcoma
   e. Given time, most lipomas will dedifferentiate into liposarcomas

29. A 40 year old female is found to have a suspected incidental left adrenal lesion on ultrasound. Which of the following CT or MR features is least likely in a phaeochromocytoma?
   a. High signal on T2-weighted images
   b. Avid enhancement post-gadolinium injection
   c. Mean lesion attenuation of more than 10 HU
   d. Less than 40% washout on delayed CT scanning
   e. Calcification

30. A 38 year old man with a swollen right hemiscrotum has an ultrasound examination. Which of the following is true?
   a. The epididymis is hypoechoic compared to the normal testis
   b. Seminomas are most commonly hyperechoic compared to the normal testis
   c. The majority of extratesticular tumours are benign
   d. Lipomas are the commonest intratesticular benign tumours
   e. Epidermoid cysts are most commonly seen in the head of the epididymis

31. A 56 year old female presents with a three-month history of pyrexia, loin pain and weight loss. Urinalysis reveals pyuria and haematuria. Urinary culture reveals *Proteus mirabilis*. A renal CT demonstrates a globally enlarged kidney with extensive perirenal inflammation, an absent nephrogram and a staghorn calculus. Which one of the following diagnoses is most likely?
   a. Leukoplakia
   b. Emphysematous pyelonephritis
   c. Pyeloureteritis cystica
   d. Xanthogranulomatous pyelonephritis
   e. Page kidney

32. A 32 year old male presents with right flank pain and an intravenous urogram is requested with the provisional diagnosis of ureteric calculi. The renal outline is smooth and wavy, with a decreased overall size. The fornices are widened with club-shaped calyces. After further questioning he reveals a recent overuse of analgesia. Which one of the following diagnoses is most likely?
   a. Acute cortical necrosis
   b. Acute tubular necrosis
   c. Papillary necrosis
   d. Acute interstitial nephritis
   e. Haemorrhagic cystitis

33. A 29 year old male has microscopic haematuria and symptoms suggesting left ureteric colic. An unenhanced CT abdomen and pelvis is requested. A 4 mm calcific density is

seen near the bladder in the left hemi-pelvis. Which one of the following signs may be useful to help differentiate between a phlebolith and ureteric calculi?
a. Lobster claw sign
b. Soft-tissue rim sign
c. Signet ring sign
d. Nubbin sign
e. Drooping lily sign

34. An 18 year old woman who is 32 weeks pregnant is referred for an obstetric ultrasound for ongoing abdominal pain. She is shown to have a small placenta relative to gestational age. Which one of the following would be a possible cause?
a. Molar pregnancy
b. Maternal diabetes
c. Umbilical vein obstruction
d. Pre-eclampsia
e. Maternal anaemia

35. A 27 year old woman who is 32 weeks pregnant is admitted with acute abdominal pain. The surgical team have requested an abdominal MRI to further investigate her pain before considering laparotomy. You are asked to protocol the request card. Which one of the following statements is correct?
a. The mother should be asked to lie prone for the scan
b. MRI should be avoided in the third trimester of pregnancy
c. Gadolinium diethylenetriaminepentaacetic acid (DTPA) chelate does not cross the placenta
d. Gadolinium-based contrast material crosses the placental membrane and circulates through the amniotic fluid
e. MRI would be the first imaging modality of choice

36. A middle-aged woman presenting to the medical team with headaches, palpitations, tachycardia and hypertension is suspected to have a phaeochromocytoma. You are asked advice on imaging modalities. Which one of the following statements is true regarding the imaging characteristics of a phaeochromocytoma?
a. I-131 MIBG imaging is only 20% sensitive for phaeochromocytoma
b. Poor contrast enhancement on CT
c. Bilateral in 25% of cases
d. Usually hypovascular on angiography
e. No change in signal intensity between in-phase and out-of-phase T1-weighted MRI images

37. A 38 year old female undergoes investigation for weight loss and abdominal fullness. CT shows large bilateral adnexal masses, ascites and several small omental soft-tissue nodules. MRI demonstrates bilateral sharply marginated ovarian tumours with preservation of the ovarian contours. The tumours consist mainly of hypointense solid material interspersed with foci of high-signal cysts. On post-contrast T1-weighted imaging the solid components are hyperintense. What is the most likely diagnosis?
a. Cystadenocarcinoma
b. Dysgerminoma
c. Krukenberg's tumour

    d. Burkitt's lymphoma

    e. Granulosa cell tumour

38. A five year old girl presents with atypical genital bleeding, breast development and pubic hair growth. T2-weighted MR imaging demonstrates a large solid mass with high signal intensity and an enlarged uterus with thick endometrium. Ascites is also present. Post-gadolinium T1-weighted imaging shows homogeneous tumour enhancement. What is the most likely diagnosis?

    a. Immature teratoma

    b. Sertoli–Leydig cell tumour

    c. Thecoma

    d. Sclerosing stromal tumour

    e. Granulosa cell tumour

39. A 23 year old female presents with acute lower abdominal pain. She has been sexually active since the age of 15 years. Ultrasound shows a well-defined, oval-shaped, relatively thin-walled, anechoic fluid-filled structure lying adjacent to the left lateral wall of the uterus. The mass appears septated although the septae do not fully cross the lumen. What is the most likely diagnosis?

    a. Hydrosalpinx

    b. Tubo-ovarian abscess

    c. Haemorrhagic ovarian cyst

    d. Endometrioma

    e. Thrombosed ovarian vein

40. A 2 cm adrenal lesion with an attenuation value of 20 HU is seen on a non-contrast CT of a patient with lung cancer. The following are all true except:

    a. A 60% washout on delayed post-contrast CT would be in keeping with an adenoma

    b. A signal intensity decrease of 40% or more on chemical shift imaging indicates malignancy

    c. PET-CT is interpreted as positive if the FDG uptake of the adrenal lesion is greater than that of the liver

    d. Functioning adrenal adenomas can be a cause for false positives on PET-CT

    e. PET-CT has somewhat higher and more consistent accuracy than dynamic CT or chemical shift MR imaging.

41. A 24 year old man is referred for an ultrasound examination following blunt trauma to the scrotum. Which of the following is not true?

    a. The left testis is more susceptible to blunt trauma

    b. Intratesticular haematomas need to be followed up until resolution

    c. Penetrating injuries are more likely to be bilateral compared to blunt injuries

    d. An ultrasound finding of an intact tunica albuginea allows the confident exclusion of a testicular rupture in the absence of a haematocoele

    e. An atrophic testis is more likely to dislocate

42. A 62 year old man presents with bilateral testicular enlargement. Ultrasound reveals bilateral smoothly enlarged testes with diffuse hypoechoic areas and normal epididymis. Which of the following is the most likely diagnosis?

    a. Lymphoma

83

    b. Metastasis from prostatic cancer

    c. Seminoma

    d. Tuberculosis

    e. Leydig cell tumour

43. A 49 year old African male presents to the outpatient urology clinic with a five-month history of macroscopic haematuria. A plain KUB X-ray is requested, which reveals thin arcuate calcification outlining the bladder and the distal ureters. Which one of the following causes is most likely?

    a. Transitional cell carcinoma

    b. Squamous cell carcinoma

    c. Schistosomiasis

    d. E. coli cystitis

    e. Proteus cystitis

44. A 21 year old female undergoes a renal ultrasound scan following an abdominal X-ray that demonstrated multiple foci of calcification in both renal areas. The ultrasound reveals multiple medullary cysts bilaterally which are seen to communicate with the collecting system. The medullae of both kidneys are of increased echogenicity. Which of the following diagnoses is most likely?

    a. Megacalicosis

    b. Multicystic dysplastic kidney

    c. Autosomal dominant polycystic kidney disease

    d. Autosomal recessive polycystic kidney disease

    e. Medullary sponge kidney

45. A 65 year old male undergoes renal CT following the finding of multiple hypoechoic masses in both kidneys on ultrasound. Multiple poorly defined masses of decreased attenuation are demonstrated, which encase the renal vessels. The vessels remain patent, however, and the renal contour is preserved. Which of the following is most likely to represent the underlying diagnosis?

    a. Renal cell carcinoma

    b. Transitional cell carcinoma

    c. Multiple myeloma

    d. Non-Hodgkin's lymphoma

    e. Reninoma

46. A routine screening mammogram of a 54 year old woman shows numerous scattered calcifications. Which of the following statements is true regarding breast calcifications?

    a. Parallel lines of calcification are usually venous in origin

    b. Malignant calcifications are usually >1 mm in size

    c. Less than 5% of microcalcifications in asymptomatic patients are associated with cancers

    d. Dermal calcifications are usually central in location

    e. Popcorn calcification is seen in fibroadenoma

47. An abdominal plain film of a four year old child taken for unexplained abdominal pain shows bilateral adrenal calcification as an incidental finding. Which of the following is the most common cause of adrenal calcification in children?

a. Wolman's disease
b. Tuberculosis
c. Adrenal haemorrhage
d. Adrenal carcinoma
e. Histoplasmosis

48. A 48 year old woman is referred to the breast clinic for investigation of a 1.5 cm lump in the right breast. Which of the following ultrasound features of a breast mass are more suggestive of a malignant than a benign pathology?
a. Acoustic shadowing
b. Anechoic contents
c. Hyperechoic pseudocapsule
d. Lack of internal blood flow on colour Doppler
e. Hypervascular surrounding tissues

49. A 13 year old girl presents with lower abdominal pain. She says she has had it intermittently for over a year. She has not yet had a period. On ultrasound examination the uterus is displaced cranially by a large cystic mass in the region of the vagina. It contains a large quantity of echogenic fluid and a fluid-debris level is visible. The bladder is not visualised. What is the most likely diagnosis?
a. Duplication cyst
b. Rectovesical fistula
c. Haematocolpos
d. Hydrometra
e. Cloacal malformation

50. A female undergoes transvaginal ultrasound for postmenopausal bleeding. In which of the following situations can you virtually exclude the presence of endometrial cancer?
a. An endometrial thickness of 5 mm in a patient who has never undergone hormone replacement therapy (HRT)
b. An endometrial thickness of 6 mm in a patient using sequential combined HRT
c. An endometrial thickness of 5 mm in a patient using continuous combined HRT
d. An endometrial thickness of 4 mm in a patient using sequential combined HRT
e. An endometrial thickness of 4 mm in a patient who has not used any form of HRT for one year or more

51. A 25 year old woman presents with an eight-month history of intermittent lower abdominal pain. Ultrasound demonstrates a 4 cm complex mass related to her left ovary. On MRI the mass has predominantly high signal on T1- and T2-weighted imaging and T2- weighted fat-suppressed sequences. The most likely diagnosis is:
a. Endometriosis
b. Follicular cyst
c. Cystadenocarcinoma
d. Dermoid cyst
e. Tubo-ovarian abscess

52. A 58 year old man presents with haematuria and suprapubic pain. Ultrasound reveals the presence of an area of bladder wall thickening and a mobile avascular mass within

the urinary bladder. A degree of right hydronephrosis is also demonstrated. Which of the following is true regarding transitional cell carcinoma (TCC)?

a. The ureter is the second commonest site of TCC after the urinary bladder
b. TCC is the most common tumour of the urinary tract
c. In the ureter, the lower ureter is the commonest site
d. It is the commonest tumour arising in the urachus
e. Previous schistosomiasis is a well-recognised risk factor

53. A 60 year old patient with a history of previous urinary tract interventions presents with right hydronephrosis and deranged renal function. Imaging suggests a mid-ureteric stenosis. An MR urogram is planned. Which of the following is true?

a. A static-fluid MR urography is performed using gadolinium-enhanced T1-weighted imaging
b. Excretory MR urogram is preferred in patients with severe renal impairment
c. T1-weighted imaging is useful in differentiating between clot and calculi
d. Renal sinus cyst can be differentiated from dilated intrarenal collecting system on T1-weighted imaging
e. Smaller filling defects are better seen on the MIP images rather than the source data

54. A 47 year old with an obstructed urinary system is advised to have a percutaneous nephrostomy. Which of the following is appropriate?

a. Persistent post-procedural haematuria usually needs a nephrectomy
b. If appropriate, the preferred site of puncture on the renal surface is just anterior to the convex lateral margin
c. A lower pole calyx is preferred when ureteral intervention is planned
d. There is a 10% chance of developing haematuria post-procedure
e. In an obstructed infected system, further imaging and manipulation are usually delayed after establishing drainage

55. A 43 year old female has a renal ultrasound which shows a left-sided renal 'mass'. The 'mass' is continuous with the renal cortex and has the same echogenicity as the cortex. It is situated at the border of the upper and mid poles of the left kidney and is seen to extend between the renal pyramids. Which one of the following are these features most likely to represent?

a. Renal scarring
b. Hypertrophied column of Bertin
c. Dromedary hump
d. Persistent fetal lobulation
e. Duplex kidney

56. A 31 year old female is admitted to hospital with placental abruption. Her renal function deteriorates significantly and therefore a renal ultrasound is requested. Kidneys with bilateral increased echogenicity and thin tramline calcification of the cortices are seen. Which of the following underlying conditions is most likely?

a. Acute cortical necrosis
b. Papillary necrosis
c. Barter syndrome
d. Drug-related nephrotoxicity
e. Renal infarction

57. A 37 year old male undergoes an intravenous urogram and the right ureter is deviated medially in the lumbar region. Which one of the following could explain this finding?
    a. Psoas muscle hypertrophy
    b. Para-aortic lymphadenopathy
    c. Retrocaval ureter
    d. Urinoma
    e. Abdominal aortic aneurysm

58. The current NHS Breast Screening Programme was set up in 1988 as a result of the Forest Report. Which one of the following statements regarding the current screening programme is correct?
    a. Screening is only available to women aged 50–70 years
    b. Women are invited to attend at two-yearly intervals
    c. It detects 15 cancers per 1000 women screened
    d. One woman per 1000 screened will be diagnosed with ductal carcinoma in situ (DCIS)
    e. Breast cancer screening has not been shown to reduce mortality from breast cancer

59. A 72 year old woman with breast cancer has the following combination of clinical and radiologic findings: a tumour measuring 3.5 cm in the right breast but with no chest wall/skin involvement; ipsilateral axillary and supraclavicular lymph node involvement with the nodes fixed to underlying structures; no internal mammary node involvement; no bone, lung or liver metastases present. Which one of the following is the correct TNM staging of her disease?
    a. T2N2M0
    b. T2N2M1
    c. T3N1M1
    d. T3N2M0
    e. T4N2M1

60. On breast MRI, which of the following features of a breast mass is more suggestive of a malignant lesion than a benign lesion?
    a. Low-signal internal septations
    b. Lobulated mass which shows no enhancement
    c. Rim-like enhancement of the mass
    d. A focal area of hypointense T2 signal adjacent to the mass
    e. Stippled enhancement

Genito-urinary, adrenal, obstetrics & gynaecology and breast – Answers

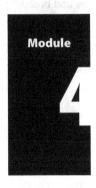

1. c. Adenomyosis
Adenomyosis is a focal or diffuse benign invasion of myometrium by endometrium, which incites reactive myometrial hyperplasia. It is associated with endometriosis (20–40%). It typically presents in multiparous women in the late reproductive years. Symptoms include pelvic pain, menorrhagia and dysmenorrhea, although adenomyosis it may be an incidental finding.

Adenomyosis may be diffuse or focal. Ultrasound appearances are variable but usually there is slight enlargement of the uterus with loss of homogeneity of the myometrium. There may be pseudo-widening of the endometrium due to increased myometrial echogenicity. MRI is more specific and demonstrates thickening of the junctional zone. When diffuse, a widened low-intensity junctional zone >12 mm confirms the diagnosis whereas <8 mm excludes the disease. For indeterminate sizes, further findings may aid the diagnosis, such as high-signal-intensity linear striations extending out from the endometrium into the myometrium on T2 and high signal foci on T1 – representing ectopic endometrial tissue/haemorrhagic foci.

When focal (adenomyoma), there is typically an oval/elongated mass with ill-defined margins residing within the myometrium which is in continuity with the junctional zone. Distinction from leiomyomas may be difficult but these tend to be round, sharply margin-ated masses occurring anywhere in the myometrium and they may contain calcifications. (Refs: Dahnert p. 1028, p. 1068; Grainger & Allison p. 1225)

2. d. T3b
Cervical neoplasms are staged according to the TNM/FIGO classification. Stage I tumours are confined to the uterus. In stage IIA, there is involvement of the upper two-thirds of the vagina. Stage IIB shows parametrial invasion without pelvic sidewall involvement. Stage IIIA demonstrates invasion into the lower third of the vagina, and IIIB includes pelvic sidewall invasion with or without hydronephrosis. Tumour invasion into the bladder and rectal mucosa or distant metastasis accounts for stage IV disease. Pelvic nodal metastases do not alter the FIGO stage but para-aortic or inguinal node metastases are classified as stage IVB. (Ref: Grainger & Allison p. 1231)

3. c. Ovarian fibroma
The condition described is Meigs syndrome. This occurs in about 1% of ovarian fibromas but is characterised by a large fibroma, ascites and a pleural effusion (typically right-sided). Ascites and effusion resolve after tumour resection.

Fibromas are benign stromal tumours composed of fibrous tissue. On ultrasound they are typically solid hypoechoic lesions with posterior acoustic enhancement.
(Ref: Bates p. 90)

4. e. Malignancy in an undescended testis
Lipoma of the cord will have a high signal on both T1-weighted and T2-weighted images. Neurofibroma will demonstrate a target sign on T2-weighted images and is of low attenuation on CT. Abscess will be clinically apparent, hypoechoic on ultrasound and have high signal on T2-weighted images. Haematomas are usually of higher attenuation on CT with varying appearances on MR, but do not demonstrate contrast enhancement.
(Ref: Bhosale PR *et al.* The inguinal canal: anatomy and imaging features of common and uncommon masses. *Radiographics* 2008; **28**: 819–835)

5. c. Corpus spongiosum enhances more rapidly following gadolinium as compared to the corpora cavernosa
Both corpus spongiosum and the corpora have a low signal on T1-weighted images and high signal on T2-weighted images. The periurethral tissue is low signal on T2-weighted images. MR cannot reliably differentiate between Buck's fascia and tunica albuginea. They are depicted as a single, thick, low-signal rim. A surface coil is used for local disease staging.
(Ref: Singh AK *et al.* Imaging of penile neoplasms. *Radiographics* 2005; **25**: 1629–1638)

6. e. Post-contrast, the peripheral zone enhances more than the central zone
The zonal anatomy is best depicted on T2-weighted images. The proximal urethra is not routinely identifiable, unless the patient is catheterised or has had previous TURP. Seminal vesicles are bright on T2-weighted images; the low-intensity structures indicate the neurovascular bundles. The peripheral zone has a higher signal on T2-weighted images and enhances more.
(Ref: Claus FG *et al.* Pretreatment evaluation of prostate cancer: role of MR imaging and 1H MR spectroscopy. *Radiographics* 2004; **24**: S167–S180)

7. d. Angiomyolipoma
The finding of fat attenuation values within a renal lesion on CT is diagnostic of angiomyolipoma. This is a benign tumour that is typically hyperechoic on ultrasound and of high signal on T1-weighted MR due to fat. It does not enhance post-gadolinium, in contrast to renal cell carcinoma, which usually does enhance.
(Ref: Dahnert p. 932)

8. a. Malakoplakia
Malakoplakia is the most likely diagnosis based on the history provided. This is a rare granulomatous infection affecting elderly females with a history of *E. coli* infections. It primarily affects the bladder, and affects the remainder of the renal tract with decreased incidence as one progresses proximally. Leukoplakia may have similar appearance, but is more common in males with bladder involvement, and is characterised by the passage of gritty soft-tissue flakes. Pyeloureteritis cystica typically produces multiple round filling defects rather than plaques.
(Ref: Grainger & Allison p. 840)

9. d. Oncocytoma
The features described are typical of renal oncocytoma. Oncocytoma is a tubular adenoma that is very rarely malignant. They are often asymptomatic even when large. The central scar is typical and is due to haemorrhage and infarction of the tumour having outgrown its

vascular supply. Radiological differentiation from renal cell carcinoma can be very difficult and percutaneous needle biopsy is unreliable. Nephrectomy is therefore often indicated.
(Ref: Grainger & Allison p. 863)

10. c. Lymphoma
Metastases to the breast are infrequent and can be difficult to distinguish from primary breast cancer. The most common primary source is lymphoma, followed by melanoma and then rhabdomyosarcoma. Most patients who are diagnosed with breast metastases already have a diagnosis of a primary tumour, however, in 25% of cases breast metastases are the first manifestation of malignancy.
(Ref: Bartella L et al. Metastases to the breast revisited: radiological-histopathological correlation. Clin Radiol 2003; 58: 524–531)

11. d. Ampullary portion of the fallopian tube
The most common site of implantation is the fallopian tube, which accounts for over 90% of ectopic pregnancies. Ovarian and abdominal sites account for only approximately 3% and 1%, respectively. Within the fallopian tube the most common site is the ampulla (73%) followed by the fimbrial and interstitial regions.
(Ref: Bouyer J et al. Sites of ectopic pregnancy: a 10 year population-based study of 1800 cases. Hum Reprod 2002; 17: 3224–3230)

12. a. Cystic adenoid malformation
The remainder of the conditions listed above will cause oligohydramnios. Polyhydramnios is defined as amniotic fluid volume >1500–2000 cm^3 at term. Most cases are due to maternal factors, with diabetes causing the majority of these. Oligohydramnios is defined as an amniotic fluid volume of <500 cm^3 at term; the most common causes include demise of the fetus, drugs and renal anomalies.
(Ref: Dahnert p. 998)

13. a. Mature cystic teratoma
Mature cystic teratomas (dermoid cysts) account for approximately 15% of all ovarian tumours. They are benign germ cell tumours containing tissues from all three germ cell layers. They most commonly present in younger women of reproductive age (20–40 years) and may be bilateral in up to 25%. They are generally cystic masses that may contain a pathognomonic distinct hyperechoic mural nodule (dermoid plug/Rokitansky nodule) which projects into the cystic lumen and causes posterior acoustic shadowing. This nodule represents in-growth of solid tissue such as hair or teeth from the tumour wall.
(Refs: Bates p. 88; Dahnert p. 1034)

14. d. Gartner duct cyst
Gartner's duct cysts are remnants of mesonephric ducts and have a reported incidence of 1–2%. They are ovoid, thin-walled cysts located at the anterolateral aspect of the upper vagina and generally measure less than 2 cm. They may contain proteinaceous material, making them slightly hyperintense on T1. They may be associated with Herlyn–Werner–Wunderlich syndrome (ipsilateral renal agenesis and ipsilateral blind vagina) and ectopic ureter inserting into the cyst.

Bartholin cysts are located at the lateral introitus adjacent to the labia minora. Nabothian cysts are epithelial inclusion cysts which develop in the endocervical canal and are most

commonly found in the perimenopausal period. Cervical fibroids and cervical polyps show mainly as solid lesions.
(Ref: Haaga p. 2085)

15. e. Endometrial polyp
Endometrial polyps are common benign tumours of the endometrial cavity. They are most common after the age of 40 years and are rare before menarche. Typical ultrasound appearance is of a hyperechoic endometrial mass which may or may not contain cystic spaces. A feeding vessel is often demonstrated from its base on power Doppler. (Submucosal fibroids are generally of reduced echogenicity).

On MRI, a mass which contains a central fibrous core that enhances post-contrast and also contains well-demarcated T2-hyperintense cysts suggests endometrial polyp. An intact junctional zone and smooth tumour-myometrium interface also favour a polyp.
(Refs: Bates p. 61; Haaga p. 2092)

16. d. Posterior urethral injuries can be seen in up to 20% of pelvic fractures in males
Urethral injuries are seen in up to 20% of male patients following pelvic fractures. They are much less common in women. The posterior urethra is the commonest site; impotence can develop in up to 40% of these patients.
(Ref: Ingram MD *et al.* Urethral injuries after pelvic trauma: evaluation with urethrography. *Radiographics* 2008; **28**: 1631–1643)

17. b. Bladder and rectal involvement are best seen on coronal images
Bladder and rectal involvement are best appreciated on axial and coronal images. MR is much more accurate for prostatic volume assessment and CT usually overestimates prostatic volume.
(Ref: Claus FG *et al.* Pretreatment evaluation of prostate cancer: role of MR imaging and 1H MR spectroscopy. *Radiographics* 2004; **24**: S167–S180)

18. a. Retroperitoneal air may indicate pulmonary injuries
Air in the retroperitoneum can follow pneumothorax. However, in the absence of pneumothorax, it is strongly indicative of duodenal/colonic injury. The posterior and anterior pararenal spaces communicate freely with the pelvic retroperitoneum, whilst the perinephric space is enclosed. The retroperitoneum is divided into three zones: I – midline retroperitoneum; II – lateral retroperitoneum; and III – pelvic retroperitoneum. Zone III is the commonest site for haematoma following blunt injury. Adrenal injuries are more common on the right. Low-attenuation fluid can be seen even in the absence of urine leak, usually indicating hypoperfusion shock syndrome.
(Ref: Daly KP *et al.* Traumatic retroperitoneal injuries: review of multidetector CT findings. *Radiographics* 2008; **28**: 1571–1590)

19. d. MRI
MRI is superior to the other imaging modalities listed at ruling out renal vein invasion. CT is still very accurate (reported as high as 96%), but MR has the advantage of being able to accurately differentiate benign from malignant thrombus. MR offers no advantage in detecting nodal disease, however, and patients being considered for curative surgery should

undergo staging CT of the chest, abdomen and pelvis. PET does not have a specific role for detecting renal vein invasion.
(Ref: Grainger & Allison p. 865)

20. a. Contrast extravasation into the paracolic gutters
Extraperitoneal rupture of the bladder is associated with pelvic fractures following trauma and cystography should be performed if this is suspected. The injury is usually at the base of the bladder, anterolaterally. Contrast is seen to extravasate with a streaky or flame-shaped appearance and collects in the space of Retzius, upper thighs, inguinal regions, perivesical fat and anterior abdominal wall. Contrast in the paracolic gutters suggests intraperitoneal rupture of the bladder. This is associated with a different method of injury, typically rupture at the bladder dome following blunt trauma with a distended bladder or secondary to iatrogenic injury such as cystoscopy.
(Ref: Dahnert p. 983)

21. e. Uniform wall thickening
The Bosniak classification groups cystic renal lesions into one of four categories based on CT/MR appearances. The differentiation between groups II and III is important as group II are typically 'follow-up lesions' and group III are 'surgical lesions'. Features of a Bosniak III lesion include irregular thickened septa, measurable enhancement, coarse irregular calcification, multiloculation, nodularity, uniform wall thickening and margin irregularity.
(Ref: Israel GM et al. Pitfalls in renal mass evaluation and how to avoid them. Radiographics 2008; 28: 1325–1338)

22. b. A crown rump length of 5 mm with no heartbeat detectable on TV scan
In order to assess the presence or absence of a heartbeat accurately on TV scanning, the crown rump length needs to be >6 mm. On TA scanning the crown rump length needs to be >10 mm in order to accurately assess the absence of a heartbeat. The other options all represent signs of fetal demise. Usually two qualified ultrasound practitioners are required to assess a fetus if there is concern regarding embryonic demise.
(Ref: Alty & Hoey p. 220)

23. d. Ductal carcinoma in situ
The most commonly associated is ductal carcinoma in situ (60%). The next most common is invasive ductal carcinoma. Fifty per cent of cases of DCIS are over 5 cm at the time of diagnosis and this often involves the nipple and subareolar ducts.
(Ref: Dahnert p. 575)

24. e. Maximum standardised uptake value >4 on FDG-PET
This is suspicious for metastatic malignant disease with the most common primary sites being lung, colon, melanoma and lymphoma. An incidental adrenal lesion is detected on 1% of abdominal CT. Even in the presence of a known malignancy, 87% of incidental lesions less than 3 cm in size are benign. Other features suggestive of malignancy are large size, irregularity and inhomogeneity.
(Refs: Dahnert p. 881; Grainger & Allison p. 1393)

25. e. Follicular cyst
These are common ovarian masses that result from a failure of the mature Graafian follicle to rupture and release ova. Typically, they are smooth, thin-walled, unilocular anechoic cysts that show spontaneous regression within four to six weeks. They may undergo haemorrhagic change producing internal echogenic material. They are generally larger than 2.5 cm and may occasionally grow up to 10 cm.
(Ref: Bates p. 80)

26. b. Ovarian torsion
Ovarian torsion usually presents in the first three decades of life and is predisposed in patients with co-existing ovarian pathology such as follicular cyst. There may be history of similar episodes indicating intermittent torsion and spontaneous detorsion. Torsion causes venous outflow obstruction and engorgement of the ovary. Eventually arterial supply is compromised and necrosis ensues.

Diagnosis is suggested by unilateral enlargement of a round or oval-shaped ovary containing multiple enlarged peripheral cysts (caused by transudation of fluid into follicles). Free fluid is present in the majority of cases. Peripheral blood flow may be present but may be absent with infarction.

Ovarian hyperstimulation can present with abdominal pain and may show an enlarged multicystic ovary associated with ascites. However, the condition usually arises from ovarian hormone stimulation in the setting of infertility. Polycystic ovary syndrome typically presents with menstrual disturbance, obesity and hyperandrogenism.
(Ref: Bates p. 85)

27. e. Ovarian volume >10 ml when no follicles measuring over 10 mm in diameter are present
Diagnosis of polycystic ovary syndrome should not be made on imaging findings alone; clinical and biochemical studies must be obtained.

The diagnosis can be supported when one or more of the following ultrasonographic features are demonstrated:

- Twelve or more follicles (3–12 mm diameter) are present in an ovary (either peripheral or diffusely arranged).
- Ovarian volume >10 ml when no follicles measuring over 10 mm in diameter are present.

If a follicle >10 mm is present then the volume should be recalculated on a repeat scan when the ovary is quiescent to prevent overestimation of the ovarian volume.
(Ref: Balen AH *et al.* Ultrasound assessment of the polycystic ovary: international consensus definitions. *Hum Reprod Update* 2003; **9**: 505–514)

28. c. Lipomas are rare in the retroperitoneum
Liposarcomas are the most common sarcomas in the retroperitoneum. Whilst well-differentiated liposarcomas are the commonest, myxomatous and dedifferentiated liposarcomas can have varying appearances and so low T1-weighted signal does not preclude a diagnosis of liposarcoma. Lipomas, whilst exceedingly rare in the retroperitoneum, almost undergo malignant changes. Whilst liposarcomas can have minimal-to-increased FDG uptake, a very FDG-avid fat-containing retroperitoneal tumour is quite likely a hibernoma.

(Ref: Craig WD *et al.* Fat-containing lesions of the retroperitoneum: radiologic-pathologic correlation. *Radiographics* 2009; **29**: 261–290)

29. e. Calcification
Whilst phaeochromocytomas can have varied appearances on CT and MR, typically they are high on T2-weighted and low on T1-weighted images and enhance avidly post-contrast. They normally have an attenuation value of more than 10 HU, but calcification is seen in only about 10% of cases.
(Ref: Blake MA *et al.* Phaeochromocytoma: an imaging chameleon. *Radiographics* 2004; **24**: S87–S99)

30. c. The majority of extratesticular tumours are benign
The epididymis is iso- or hyperechoic compared to the testis. Seminomas are homogenous masses and hypoechoic to the testis. Epidermoid cysts are the commonest intratesticular benign neoplasm. Lipomas are the commonest benign tumours in the spermatic cord.
(Ref: Kim *et al.* US MR imaging correlation in pathologic conditions of the scrotum. *Radiographics* 2007; **27**: 1239–1253)

31. d. Xanthogranulomatous pyelonephritis
The most likely diagnosis is xanthogranulomatous pyelonephritis. This is a chronic granulomatous infection in a chronically obstructed kidney, often secondary to a staghorn calculus. It often presents insidiously in middle-aged to elderly females. It is most commonly diffuse, but the focal form seen in 15% of cases may provide a diagnostic dilemma as it can be difficult to confidently distinguish from renal cell carcinoma.
(Ref: Dahnert p. 702)

32. c. Papillary necrosis
Papillary necrosis occurs due to ischaemic damage to the medulla of the kidney, and does not primarily involve the cortex. There are many causes including diabetes, analgesic nephropathy, pyelonephritis, renal vein thrombosis and sickle cell disease. It may be localised or diffuse, bilateral or unilateral depending on the cause. Intravenous urogram appearances are varied and include clubbed calyces, calcification and sloughing of necrotic papilla and alteration in the renal contour.
(Ref: Chapman & Nakielny 2003 p. 338)

33. b. Soft-tissue rim sign
The soft-tissue rim sign is thickening of the ureteric wall around the calculus due to oedema. It has a reported specificity of up to 92% for renal calculi. Other signs that may favour a diagnosis of ureteric calculi include asymmetrical perinephric fat stranding, periureteral oedema, hydronephrosis and unilateral renal enlargement. The lobster claw and signet ring signs concern papillary necrosis on intravenous urogram. The nubbin and drooping lily signs both refer to ureteral duplication.
(Ref: Zagoria p. 188)

34. d. Pre-eclampsia
Pre-eclampsia, IUGR, chromosomal abnormality and intrauterine infection can all cause a decrease in placental size. Enlargement of the placenta is defined as a measurement of

>5 cm when obtained at right angles to the long axis of the placenta. The causes of placentomegaly include maternal diabetes, chronic intrauterine infection (e.g. syphilis), maternal anaemia, thalassaemia and twin–twin transfusion syndrome. Fetal chromosomal abnormalities may cause either a large or small placenta.
(Ref: Dahnert p. 999)

35. d. Gadolinium-based contrast material crosses the placental membrane and circulates through the amniotic fluid

The use of MRI in the evaluation of abdominal pain in pregnant patients is increasing. The primary imaging modality of choice, however, remains ultrasound, and MRI is usually reserved for situations where the ultrasound findings are equivocal. The use of gadolinium is not usually necessary in the investigation of abdominal pain in the acute setting and there is little evidence as to its effect on the fetus.
(Refs: Baughman WC *et al.* Placenta accreta: spectrum of US and MR imaging findings. *Radiographics* 2008; **28**: 1905–1916; Pedrosa I *et al.* MR imaging of acute right lower quadrant pain in pregnant and nonpregnant patients. *Radiographics* 2007; **27**: 721–743)

36. e. No change in signal intensity between in-phase and out-of-phase T1-weighted MRI images

There is no change between the in-phase and out-of-phase imaging on MRI as there is very low fat content in phaeochromocytoma. MR is the method of choice for imaging and usually (60%) the phaeochromocytoma will be hyperintense to spleen on T2-weighted imaging. Angiography can localise the lesion in >90% of cases. Appearance on ultrasound can be variable with about 70% appearing as solid lesions whilst 15% are cystic. The 'rule of tens' applies to phaeochromocytoma, i.e. 10% are bilateral, 10% are extra-adrenal, 10% are malignant and 10% are familial.
(Ref: Dahnert p. 944)

37. c. Krukenberg's tumour

Krukenburg's tumours are metastatic tumours of the ovary. The colon and stomach are the most common primary tumour sites, but other sites, such as the breast, lung and pancreas, have also been reported. They display characteristic imaging features, including bilateral, sharply marginated oval tumours which preserve the contour of the ovary. Identification of hypointense solid components on T2-weighted imaging corresponding to areas of dense collagenous stroma is also considered characteristic.
(Ref: Ha HK *et al.* Krukenberg's tumor of the ovary: MR imaging features. *AJR Am J Roentgenol* 1995; **164**: 1435–1439)

38. e. Granulosa cell tumour

Granulosa cell tumours are the most common ovarian tumours with oestrogenic manifestations that are classified as sex-cord-stromal tumours. They are subdivided into adult and juvenile types. The juvenile form affects prepubertal children and causes pseudoprecocity. In about a third of cases Sertoli–Leydig cell tumours cause virilisation. Thecomas are oestrogen-producing tumours but more than 80% occur in postmenopausal women. Immature teratomas are extremely rare but do occur in children. Elevated alpha-fetoprotein is found in up to 65% of cases. Sclerosing stromal tumours usually affect women younger than 30 years of age and a few cases have shown androgenic or oestrogenic manifestations.

They are also known as hypervascular tumours which show early peripheral enhancement with centripetal progression.
(Ref: Tanaka YO *et al.* Functioning ovarian tumors: direct and indirect findings at MR imaging. *Radiographics* 2004; **24**: S147–S166)

39. a. Hydrosalpinx
Hydrosalpinx describes a fallopian tube filled with fluid. The fluid is most often anechoic. When the fluid becomes infected, the term pyosalpinx is used and the fluid contents tend to be echogenic. Hydro/pyosalpinx appear as tortuous, well-defined, fluid-filled, oval-shaped structures which extend from the cornua to the ovaries. They are often mistaken for multicystic adnexal masses or septated ovarian cysts due to apparent internal septations. However, the septa, actually the folded wall of the fallopian tube, do not cross the lumen completely. Hydro/pyosalpinx occur most commonly as a result of acute salpingitis and pelvic inflammatory disease (history of early sexual activity/multiple sexual partners). They have also been reported following pelvic surgery.

Tubo-ovarian abscesses tend to be multilocular, irregular, thick-walled, complex masses containing debris and internal septations. Internal fluid-fluid levels or gas may also be seen.
(Refs: Bates p. 108; Dahnert p. 1058)

40. b. A signal intensity decrease of 40% or more on chemical shift imaging indicates malignancy
A signal intensity decrease of less than 20% is usually indicative of malignancy in an adrenal lesion.
(Ref: Chong S *et al.* Integrated PET-CT for the characterization of adrenal gland lesions in cancer patients: diagnostic efficacy and interpretation pitfalls. *Radiographics* 2006; **26**: 1811–1826)

41. a. The left testis is more susceptible to blunt trauma
The testis suffers blunt trauma against the thigh or the symphysis pubis and the right testis, being higher, is more susceptible. Intratesticular haematomas should be followed up to resolution to rule out an underlying neoplasm and also rule out any ensuing complications such as abscess formation which may necessitate orchidectomy.
(Ref: Bhatt S *et al.* Role of US in testicular and scrotal trauma. *Radiographics* 2008; **28**: 1617–1629)

42. a. Lymphoma
This is the wrong age group for Leydig cell tumour (childhood) and seminoma (around 40 years). Lymphoma is the commonest tumour in this age group. It is more likely to have a diffuse hypoechoic appearance and be bilateral as compared to metastasis, which usually presents with multiple focal lesions. Tuberculosis of the testis is most often secondary to epididymitis.
(Ref: Dahnert p. 978)

43. c. Schistosomiasis
The differential for bladder calcification includes tuberculosis, post-radiotherapy cystitis, urachal carcinoma, TCC, and squamous cell carcinoma. However, schistosomiasis is the commonest cause, especially in the African population, where it is often endemic. The

bladder is usually a normal size and shape, with thin curvilinear calcifications. Ureteric strictures, inflammatory pseudopolyps and vesicoureteric reflux are seen in addition to bladder and ureteric calcification.
(Ref: Chapman & Nakielny 2003 p. 350)

44. e. Medullary sponge kidney
The features are those of medullary sponge kidney. This is a non-inheritable condition that produces cystic dilatation of the collecting ducts and nephrocalcinosis; 75% of cases are bilateral and it is usually asymptomatic. It is associated with an increased incidence of infection and urolithiasis but is not thought to predispose to malignancy.
(Refs: Chapman & Nakielny 2003 p. 314; Dahnert p. 935)

45. d. Non-Hodgkin's lymphoma
The most likely diagnosis is non-Hodgkin's lymphoma. Primary renal involvement is rare, but is often involved either by haematogenous spread or direct invasion. The kidneys represent one of the most common extra-nodal sites of disease in non-Hodgkin's lymphoma, but are rarely involved in Hodgkin's disease. Involvement is usually bilateral, with masses of decreased attenuation and mild homogenous enhancement with intravenous contrast on CT. Patency of the renal vessels despite encasement is highly suggestive, as is preservation of the normal renal contour.
(Ref: Silverman & Cohan p. 127)

46. e. Popcorn calcification is seen in fibroadenoma
Popcorn calcification is pathognomonic for fibroadenoma. The majority of biopsied clusters of calcifications represent a benign process (75–80%). Malignant calcifications are usually small (<0.5 mm) and are usually irregular in size and density. They are, however, usually closely grouped. Benign calcifications tend to be numerous and scattered throughout the breast.
(Ref: Dahnert p. 547)

47. c. Adrenal haemorrhage
All of the above cause adrenal calcification. The most common cause in both adults and children is adrenal haemorrhage. In adults this is most commonly unilateral and right-sided. In children adrenal haemorrhage is most common in newborn infants and is induced by episodes of birth trauma or hypoxia, but may also be related to non-accidental injury. Wolman's disease is a rare disease causing enlarged calcified adrenal glands, hepatomegaly and splenomegaly.
(Ref: Brant & Helms pp. 774–775)

48. a. Acoustic shadowing
Acoustic shadowing along with ill-defined margins, surrounding architectural distortion, heterogeneous internal echoes and a height measurement greater than width measurement (with the transducer parallel to the longitudinal axis) are all features more suggestive of a malignant rather than a benign pathology. A hypoechoic lesion containing echogenic debris along with lack of internal blood flow and hypervascularity of surrounding tissues are in keeping with a breast abscess.
(Ref: Stavros AT et al. Solid breast nodules: use of sonography to distinguish between benign and malignant lesions. Radiology 1995; 196: 123–134)

49. c. Haematocolpos

Haematocolpos is the accumulation of blood within the vagina and is typically caused by an imperforated hymen. This causes acute-on-chronic lower abdominal/pelvic pain as menstrual blood is prevented from normal discharge (apparent lack of menstruation). Ultrasound reveals an echogenic cystic mass with or without fluid-debris levels in the region of the vagina. The distended vagina often causes displacement of the uterus and compression of the bladder so that the latter may not be visualised.

Cloacal malformation is a single perineal orifice for the bladder, vagina and rectum caused by early embryonic arrest. It manifests in the newborn period. Hydrometra is fluid within the uterus and may be due to cervical or vaginal dysgenesis. Rectal duplication cysts may reveal an echogenic cystic mass in childhood but they often present with constipation and faecal soiling.

(Ref: Bates p. 117; Dahnert p. 1046)

50. d. An endometrial thickness of 4 mm in a patient using sequential combined HRT

An endometrial thickness of 3 mm can be used to exclude endometrial cancer in women who:

- Have never used HRT, or
- Have not used any form of HRT for $\geq$ one year, or
- Are using continuous combined HRT.

In the above conditions the post-test risk of a patient having endometrial cancer is 0.6–0.8% when the endometrial thickness is 3 mm but 20–22% when the endometrial thickness is >3 mm.

An endometrial thickness of 5 mm can be used to exclude endometrial cancer in women using sequential combined HRT (or having used it within the past year). In this scenario the post-test risk of a patient having endometrial cancer is 0.1–0.2% when the endometrial thickness is 5 mm but 2–5% when the endometrial thickness is >5 mm.

(Ref: Scottish Intercollegiate Guidelines Network. *Investigation of Post-menopausal Women.* September 2002. http://www.sign.ac.uk/guidelines/fulltext/61/index.html)

51. a. Endometriosis

The ovaries are the most common site for endometriosis, accounting for greater than 80%. Other sites include the uterosacral ligaments, pouch of Douglas, uterine serosal surface, fallopian tubes and rectosigmoid.

MRI is more specific than either CT or ultrasound in its detection. Typically, MR demonstrates a homogeneously hyperintense cyst due to the presence of methaemoglobin, which shortens T1. It is also hyperintense on fat-suppressed T2-weighted imaging, which virtually excludes a dermoid cyst. On T2-weighted imaging there may be faint or complete loss of signal. This phenomenon is referred to as 'shading' and results from the high protein and iron concentration from recurrent haemorrhage into the endometrioma.

(Ref: Kuligowska E *et al.* Pelvic pain: overlooked and underdiagnosed gynecologic conditions. *Radiographics* 2005; **25**: 3–20)

52. b. TCC is the most common tumour of the urinary tract

TCC is the commonest cancer in the urinary tract. Whilst a predominant majority of them develop in the bladder, the renal pelvis is the second commonest site. In the ureter, the

upper ureter is the commonest site. Adenocarcinoma is the commonest tumour in the urinary tract. Schistosomiasis is associated with squamous cell carcinoma.
(Ref: Dahnert p. 979)

53.   c. T1-weighted imaging is useful in differentiating between clot and calculi
A static-fluid MR urogram is a heavily T2-weighted technique similar to MRCP. Excretory urogram is a post-gadolinium injection T1-weighted technique. A static-fluid MR urogram is preferred in patients with renal failure. Renal sinus cysts cannot often be differentiated from dilated intrarenal collecting systems on T1-weighted and T2-weighted images. They are better appreciated on the excretory urogram. Source data should be reviewed to ensure that small filling defects are not missed.
(Ref: Leyendecker JR *et al.* MR urography: techniques and clinical applications. *Radiographics* 2008; **28**: 23–46)

54.   e. In an obstructed infected system, further imaging and manipulation are usually delayed after establishing drainage
The most common reasons for persistent haematuria are traumatic arteriovenous fistula, pseudoaneurysm or vascular injury, all of which are usually managed endovascularly. Brodel's avascular plane is just posterior to the convex lateral margin. Whilst an easily accessible lower pole calyx is usually the target for a simple nephrostomy drainage, for ureteral interventions, a posterior calyx in the mid or upper polar region may be better. Almost all patients develop haematuria, but 1–3% may need transfusion or further intervention.
(Ref: Dyer RB *et al.* Percutaneous nephrostomy with extensions of the technique: step by step. *Radiographics* 2002; **22**: 503–525)

55.   b. Hypertrophied column of Bertin
Many lesions may be mistaken for a renal cell carcinoma on imaging, and it is important to be able to differentiate such 'pseudotumours' from genuine carcinomas. The features described in the question are consistent with a prominent column of Bertin. This is normal renal tissue located between the pyramids and extending into the renal sinus. The key features include continuity with the cortex, identical echogenicity to normal cortex and the lack of mass effect or renal outline deformity. A dromedary hump is a focal bulge on the lateral border of the left kidney caused by its relationship with the adjacent spleen. Persistent fetal lobulation can be identified by indentations of the renal surface that overlie the space between the pyramids, whereas renal scarring lies directly over the medullary pyramids.
(Ref: Bhatt *et al.* Renal pseudotumors. *AJR Am J Roentgenol* 2007; **188**: 1380–1387)

56.   a. Acute cortical necrosis
The features described are typical of cortical nephrocalcinosis. Causes of cortical nephrocalcinosis include acute cortical necrosis, chronic glomerulonephritis, sickle cell disease, Alport syndrome and congenital oxalosis. Acute cortical necrosis is a rare cause of acute renal failure, and is most commonly due to complications of pregnancy such as placental abruption, infected abortion and severe eclampsia.
(Refs: Dahnert p. 916; DeCherney & Nathan p. 424)

57. c. Retrocaval ureter

Medial deviation of the ureter is seen with retrocaval ureter on the right side and with retroperitoneal fibrosis. The other conditions listed all cause medial deviation of the ureter in the lumbar region. Retrocaval ureter is a rare entity which is caused by abnormal embryogenesis of the IVC. There may be symptoms of right ureteral obstruction and recurrent urinary tract infections.
(Ref: Dahnert p. 896, p. 970)

58. d. One woman per 1000 screened will be diagnosed with ductal carcinoma in situ (DCIS)

In the 2007–2008 review statistics, eight cancers were detected per 1000 women screened. Women between the ages of 50 and 70 years are invited to attend the Breast Cancer Screening Programme at three-yearly intervals. However, women over the age of 70 are encouraged to make their own appointments to attend. The IARC working group, comprising 24 experts from 11 countries, evaluated all the available evidence on breast screening and determined that there is a 35% reduction in mortality from breast cancer among screened women aged 50–69 years. This means that out of every 500 women screened, one life will be saved.
(Refs: IARC. *7th Handbook on Cancer Prevention.* Lyons: IARC, 2002; National Health Service. *NHS Breast Screening Programme Audit 2007–8.* London: NHS, 2009)

59. b. T2N2M1

The correct TNM staging is T2N2M1. The presence of involved ipsilateral supraclavicular nodes makes the staging M1 even in the absence of other distant metastases. T2 tumours encompass those which are more than 2 cm but less than 5 cm in diameter. N2 disease signifies involved axillary nodes which are fixed either to one another or to underlying structures. N3 disease signifies internal mammary involvement.
(Ref: Barter S, Lyburn I. *RITI ELD 4a_015 Staging of Breast Cancer and Metastatic Disease.*

60. c. Rim-like enhancement of the mass

Rim-like enhancement is a relatively rare finding, but has a high correlation with malignancy (positive predictive value 84%). A focal area of hyperintense signal on T2 near a lesion is highly suggestive of malignancy. Whilst the other characteristics may be present in a malignant lesion, all are more suggestive of benign pathology. Irregular spiculated margins of a mass have a high positive predictive value for malignancy. Other features suggestive of malignancy are heterogenous internal septations and enhancing internal septa.
(Ref: Macura KJ *et al.* Patterns of enhancement on breast MR images: interpretation and imaging pitfalls. *Radiographics* 2006; **26**: 1719–1734)

Paediatric – Questions

1. A ten year old boy complaining of generalised back pain is referred by his GP for a thoracic spine plain film which shows anterior vertebral body scalloping. Which of the following would be a cause of anterior vertebral body scalloping?
   a. Neurofibromatosis
   b. Acromegaly
   c. Achondroplasia
   d. Ehlers–Danlos syndrome
   e. Down's syndrome

2. A ten day old baby is referred for a hip ultrasound as clinical examination has revealed a 'clicky' right hip. Which of the following parameters is reassuring for a normal hip joint?
   a. Alpha angle >60°
   b. Alpha angle <60°
   c. Beta angle >77°
   d. 25% coverage of the femoral head
   e. Acetabular angle >30°

3. A two week old neonate presents with central cyanosis and respiratory distress. Plain chest radiograph reveals pulmonary plethora. Which is the most likely underlying congenital heart disease?
   a. VSD
   b. Tetralogy of Fallot
   c. PDA
   d. Pulmonary stenosis
   e. Total anomalous pulmonary venous return (TAPVC)

4. A 16 year old presents with recurrent pneumothoraces. Past history reveals the presence of a lytic lesion of the parietal bone with a tender soft-tissue mass. Which of the following features is most likely seen on HRCT?
   a. Evenly distributed smooth thin-walled cysts
   b. Centrilobular nodules
   c. Extensive paraseptal emphysema with bulla formation
   d. Sparing of the apices
   e. Cystic lesions along the course of the bronchial tree

5. A ten year old boy presents with a history of progressive gait abnormalities. Plain radiographs of the thoraco-lumbar spine show widening of the spinal canal at T8-L1. MRI demonstrates an eccentric, ill-defined, homogeneous intramedullary lesion which

is hypointense to the cord on T1 and hyperintense on T2. There is patchy, irregular enhancement post-contrast. What is the most likely diagnosis?

a. Lipoma
b. Ependymoma
c. Astrocytoma
d. Ganglioglioma
e. Haemangioblastoma

6. A two year old girl presents with recurrent headaches, neck pain and vomiting. She is found to have kyphoscoliosis and café-au-lait spots. CT brain shows a mostly cystic mass within the right cerebellar hemisphere. There is some calcification. After contrast, there is enhancement of the cystic wall and strong enhancement of a mural nodule. The most likely diagnosis is:

a. Haemangioblastoma
b. Medulloblastoma
c. Metastasis
d. Pilocytic astrocytoma
e. Arachnoid cyst

7. A neonate has an abdominal ultrasound following the finding of a palpable abdominal mass. The right kidney is normal. The left kidney is replaced by multiple cysts of varying size and shape. There is no communication between the cysts, which are separated by septae. Which of the following is the most likely diagnosis?

a. Multilocular cystic renal tumour
b. Autosomal recessive polycystic kidney disease
c. Autosomal dominant polycystic kidney disease
d. Multicystic dysplastic kidney
e. Medullary sponge kidney

8. A three year old boy has an ultrasound and an abdominal CT scan following the discovery of a palpable abdominal mass. No other symptoms are present. A large abdominal mass measuring 9 cm in maximum cross-sectional dimensions is seen. Which one of the following features would favour a diagnosis of Wilms tumour rather than neuroblastoma?

a. Calcification
b. Bone metastases
c. Lung metastases
d. Encasement of the major vessels
e. Displacement of the kidney

9. A ten year old boy presents with severe localised pain in the distal femur with an associated swelling. Blood films show a leucocytosis and anaemia. At the time of diagnosis he has both lung and bone metastases. The most likely diagnosis is:

a. Osteosarcoma
b. Giant cell tumour
c. Lymphoma
d. Ewing's sarcoma
e. Clear cell sarcoma

10. A plain film taken of a five year old boy following a fall shows a fracture of the distal radius. The fracture runs through the physis and the metaphysis, but the epiphysis is not involved. The correct classification of this fracture is:
    a. Salter Harris I
    b. Salter Harris II
    c. Salter Harris III
    d. Salter Harris IV
    e. Greenstick fracture

11. A ten year old girl falls and injures her left elbow. No bony injury is demonstrated on plain radiographs. On interpretation of the plain radiographs, which one of the following ossification centres is the least likely to be present?
    a. Trochlear
    b. Radial head
    c. Medial epicondyle
    d. Lateral epicondyle
    e. Olecranon

12. A four year old girl presents with persistent left upper lobe pneumonia with a finger-like opacity projecting from the hilum. The most likely diagnosis is:
    a. Bronchial atresia
    b. Intralobar sequestration
    c. Staphylococcal pneumonia
    d. Congenital lobar emphysema
    e. Bronchogenic cyst

13. A five month old baby presents with failure to thrive and respiratory distress. Plain radiograph demonstrates a left basal homogenous opacity devoid of air broncho-grams. Which of the following is least likely on further imaging?
    a. Radionuclide angiography does not demonstrate perfusion in the pulmonary phase
    b. Invested in its own pleura
    c. Co-existing anomalies are common
    d. It is usually supplied by branches from the descending aorta
    e. Commonly drains into the left atrium

14. A 14 year old patient with Turner syndrome presents with severe headache. Clinical examination confirms upper limb hypertension and a murmur. Which of the following signs is likely on the plain films?
    a. Boot-shaped heart
    b. Snowman sign
    c. Figure-of-three sign
    d. Egg-on-a-string sign
    e. Scimitar sign

15. An 11 year old boy undergoes investigation for a mass in his right orbit. CT shows a hypodense mass located in the upper temporal quadrant. The Hounsfield units are positive throughout the lesion. There is no calcification and the lesion does not enhance. There is adjacent scalloping of the lateral orbital wall. On MRI, the lesion is

hypointense on T1 and hyperintense on T2, FLAIR and diffusion-weighted imaging. What is the most likely diagnosis?

a. Orbital teratoma
b. Orbital pseudotumour
c. Conjunctival choristoma
d. Dermoid cyst
e. Epidermoid cyst

16. The mother of a three week old child notices a mass in her baby's lower neck. The child is otherwise well. There is a history of normal pregnancy and the child was delivered by forceps. Ultrasound scan reveals homogeneous enlargement of the lower third of the right sternocleidomastoid muscle but no focal lesion is identified. T2-weighted MRI shows diffuse abnormal high signal intensity over the same area. The most likely diagnosis is:

a. Haematoma
b. Branchial cleft cyst
c. Fibromatosis colli
d. Neuroblastoma
e. Cystic hygroma

17. A three year old boy presents with headaches and drowsiness. Examination reveals papilloedema. CT brain shows hydrocephalus and a mildly hyperdense homogeneous mass at the trigone of the left lateral ventricle. There is intense homogeneous enhancement post-contrast. On MRI the lesion is slightly hyperintense on T1 and slightly hypointense on T2-weighted imaging relative to white matter. Gadolinium injection confirms an intraventricular enhancing tumour island. The most likely diagnosis is:

a. Choroid plexus papilloma
b. Intraventricular meningioma
c. Ependymoma
d. Cavernous angioma
e. Pilocytic astrocytoma

18. An eight month old girl is diagnosed with neuroblastoma following the finding of an abdominal mass. At CT the tumour is found to arise from the right suprarenal region and does not cross the midline. There are liver metastases, and bone marrow aspirates are positive for tumour. However, there is no evidence of skeletal metastases on plain films. What is the correct stage of the tumour?

a. Stage I
b. Stage II
c. Stage III
d. Stage IV
e. Stage IVs

19. A two year old boy presents with failure to thrive and a left-sided abdominal mass is found. An ultrasound scan reveals a left-sided hydronephrosis. The right kidney is normal. Which one of the following is most likely to be found as the underlying cause?

a. Posterior urethral valve
b. Pelvic–ureteric junction obstruction

c. Urethral diverticulum

d. Ureteric calculus

e. Ureterocoele

20. A neonatal boy has a renal ultrasound performed for the investigation of urinary obstructive symptoms. The ultrasound shows a distended urinary bladder with bilateral hydronephrosis. Which one of the following is the most likely underlying pathology?

a. Posterior urethral valve

b. Neurogenic bladder

c. Horseshoe kidney

d. Ectopic ureterocoeles

e. Urethral diverticulum

21. In a neonatal lumbar spine film showing a 'bone-within-bone' appearance, which of the following would NOT be a plausible explanation?

a. Osteopetrosis

b. Normal variant

c. Congenital syphilis

d. Sickle cell anaemia

e. Achondroplasia

22. A six year old boy presents to A&E with pain in the right hip and knee, limitation of movement and a limp. Plain radiographs show flattening of the capital femoral epiphysis and enlargement of the medial joint space. Blood tests are normal. Which of the following is the most likely diagnosis?

a. Legg–Calve–Perthes disease

b. Transient synovitis

c. Osteomyelitis

d. Slipped upper femoral epiphysis

e. Developmental dysplasia of the hip

23. A two year old boy is brought to the A&E department with a history of falling down the stairs. There is some concern regarding the delay in presentation and the consistency of the history. Bruising is noted to various parts of the child's body. A skeletal survey is performed as there is concern regarding non-accidental injury. Which of the following findings would be the most concerning for non-accidental injury?

a. Salter Harris II fracture to the distal radius

b. Spiral fracture of the tibia

c. Scapula fracture

d. Linear parietal skull fracture

e. Avulsion of the medial epicondyle

24. A 12 year old girl with developmental delay undergoes a skeletal radiograph for assessment of bone age. Plain films of her hands show granular fragmented epiphyses, and bone age is calculated as 9.5 years. Which one of the following is the most likely diagnosis?

a. Pseudohypoparathyroidism

b. Hypothyroidism

    c. McCune–Albright syndrome
    d. Hyperthyroidism
    e. Acrodysostosis

25. A 14 year old with thalassaemia presents with mild breathlessness. The only abnormality on the chest radiograph is a well-rounded opacity without any air bronchograms. The likely location would be:
    a. Perihilar
    b. Anterior mediastinal
    c. Abutting the chest wall
    d. Paravertebral
    e. Apical

26. A four year old child with a known malignancy presents with multiple pulmonary metastases. Which of the following is the most likely radiological description of the primary lesion?
    a. CT of the abdomen demonstrating a large mass in the left flank displacing the kidney inferiorly with stippled calcification
    b. CT of the abdomen demonstrating a large low-attenuation hepatic mass pre-contrast which demonstrates early and avid enhancement post-contrast
    c. CT of the abdomen demonstrating a low-attenuation hepatic mass with rim enhancement
    d. Plain radiograph of the right femur revealing a moth-eaten permeative lesion
    e. A well-circumscribed heterogeneous mass in the left kidney which enhances to a lesser degree than the kidney

27. A neonate presents with respiratory distress a week after birth. Plain radiograph demonstrates a hazy opacity in the left upper zone. Follow-up radiograph a few days later demonstrates clearing up of the opacity noted previously and a hyperlucent underlying lung with evidence of a contralateral shift. Which of the following is not a likely cause for the findings?
    a. Bronchial dysplasia
    b. Inspissated mucous
    c. Patent ductus arteriosus
    d. Anomalous origin of the right subclavian artery
    e. Bronchial web

28. A neonate presenting with respiratory distress and a scaphoid abdomen is diagnosed with congenital diaphragmatic hernia following imaging. Which of the following is true?
    a. Right-sided hernia is frequently fatal
    b. The anterior hernias are larger
    c. The stomach is the commonest viscera to herniate
    d. Morgagni hernia present earlier
    e. Early intrauterine diagnosis is associated with an improved prognosis

29. A two month old child is brought to hospital as his parents have noticed he has become more floppy over the preceding weeks. Examination reveals marked hypotonia, head lag and increased head circumference (>98th percentile). CT brain shows low-density white matter. T2-weighted MRI demonstrates diffuse, symmetric increased signal

intensity throughout the white matter. There is relative sparing of the internal and external capsules and also the corpus callosum. Both globus pallidi show high signal intensity but there is relative sparing of the putamen and caudate nucleus. Which of the following would fail to confirm the diagnosis?

a. Brain biopsy
b. Proton MR spectroscopy
c. Quantitative urine study
d. Fibroblast cultures
e. Diffusion-weighted MRI

30. An 18 month old boy is investigated for hyperactivity and laughing fits. MRI demonstrates a lesion arising near the floor of the third ventricle, posterior to the pituitary infundibulum. It projects into the suprasellar cistern. The lesion is isointense to grey matter on T1- and T2-weighted imaging and does not enhance following gadolinium administration. The most likely diagnosis is:

a. Germinoma
b. Pituitary adenoma
c. Hypothalamic hamartoma
d. Rathke's cleft cyst
e. Langerhans' cell histiocytosis

31. A ten year old girl attends the emergency department after a head injury. You are requested to perform an acute CT scan of her head. According to NICE guidelines for head injury, which one of the following criteria alone does not warrant an acute head CT scan?

a. Retrograde amnesia lasting >5 minutes
b. Antegrade amnesia lasting >5 minutes
c. More than one episode of vomiting
d. CSF otorrhea
e. Abnormal drowsiness

32. A three year old boy presents with seizures and headaches. CT head shows a hypoattenuating mass lying superior to the lateral ventricles, within the frontal region. It displays negative Hounsfield units and peripheral calcification but does not enhance. There is partial agenesis of the corpus callosum. MRI of the brain demonstrates a pericallosal tumour which is hyperintense on T1 and less hyperintense on T2-weighted imaging. What is the most likely diagnosis?

a. Dermoid tumour
b. Lipoma
c. Teratoma
d. Neurocytoma
e. Ependymoma

33. A neonate is found to have hypotonic abdominal wall musculature, and further investigations reveal bowel malrotation and cryptorchidism. Which of the following conditions is most likely?

a. Prune belly syndrome
b. Zellweger syndrome
c. Wolman disease

d. Meckel–Gruber syndrome

e. Wunderlich syndrome

34. A two month old boy born prematurely has a CT abdomen following macroscopic haematuria and a palpable abdominal mass. A large intrarenal mass is seen, which replaces the majority of the renal parenchyma, involves the renal sinus and does not display any venous extension, collecting system involvement or calcification. Which one of the following diagnoses is most likely?

a. Metanephric adenoma

b. Mesoblastic nephroma

c. Wilms tumour

d. Nephroblastomatosis

e. Neuroblastoma

35. A premature neonate presents with bilious vomiting in the first few days of life. A plain abdominal X-ray shows prominent gas-fluid levels in the duodenal bulb and in the gastric fundus. There is absence of gas in the remainder of the small and large bowel. Which one of the following diagnoses is most likely?

a. Choledochal cyst

b. Annular pancreas

c. Duodenal atresia

d. Duodenal duplication cyst

e. Ladd bands

36. A young boy presents with abdominal pain and vomiting. Ultrasound of the abdomen confirms ileocolic intussusception. Which one of the following features is associated with a good chance of successful hydrostatic reduction?

a. Symptom history of greater than 48 hours

b. Small bowel obstruction

c. Presence of blood flow within the intussusceptum

d. Passage of blood per rectum

e. Age less than three months

37. A seven year old boy presents to the minor injuries unit following a minor fall five weeks earlier. He complains of pain around the left elbow joint and has a limited range of movement. Blood tests are normal. Plain film of the elbow shows a small joint effusion and fragmentation of the capitellar epiphysis. Which one of the following is the most likely diagnosis?

a. Osteochondrosis of the capitellum (Panner's disease)

b. Osteomyelitis

c. Osteochondritis dessicans

d. Juvenile chronic arthritis

e. Osteochondral capitellum fracture

38. A 13 year old girl is noted to have a curvature to her spine. Plain radiographs confirm the presence of a scoliosis with a convexity to the right. The most likely cause of this would be:

a. Neurofibromatosis

b. Idiopathic

c. Segmental abnormality
d. Osteoid osteoma
e. Infection

39. A 12 year old boy attends A&E after falling off his bike. He complains of pain in the right hand. Plain radiographs show no bony injury. However, a small well-rounded lesion is seen in the proximal phalanx of the index finger. This has a ground glass appearance and contains dystrophic calcifications. There is no cortical breakthrough or periosteal reaction. The most likely cause of this lesion is:
a. Simple bone cyst
b. Aneurysmal bone cyst
c. Enchondroma
d. Epidermoid inclusion cyst
e. Fibrous dysplasia

40. A 15 year old girl referred for a chest radiograph demonstrates a large well-rounded mediastinal mass. CT suggests a teratoma. Which of the following is true?
a. They are often inseparable from the thymus
b. They are always anterior mediastinal
c. Rim enhancement indicates malignancy
d. A fat-fluid level is a common and specific sign
e. Homogenous soft-tissue density precludes a diagnosis of teratoma

41. A seven year old girl with repeated chest infections and chronic cough presents with another episode of acute exacerbation. She is known to have raised sodium and chloride in her sweat. Which of the following features is least likely on an HRCT of her chest?
a. Cylindrical bronchiectasis
b. Centrilobular emphysema
c. Segmental/subsegmental atelectasis
d. Branching intrabronchial soft tissue
e. Hilar lymphadenopathy

42. An abdominal CT in a neonate with major congenital abnormalities demonstrates a large central liver and absence of spleen. Which of the following features is likely on chest CT?
a. Absence of the minor fissure on the right
b. Hyparterial bronchus on the right
c. Presence of three lobes on the left
d. Tubular appendages bilaterally
e. Absence of SVC

43. A teenage boy with a history of nasal speech is investigated for recurrent severe epistaxis. The ear, nose and throat surgeon suggests the possibility of a juvenile angiofibroma. Which of the following CT findings would you consider typical for this lesion?
a. A highly vascular nasal mass causing widening of the pterygopalatine fissure
b. A relatively avascular fibrous nasal mass centred over Little's area
c. A vascular mass centred over the pterygopalatine fossa best demonstrated on delayed imaging

d. A fibrous mass extending posteriorly into the middle cranial fossa with relatively little bone erosion

e. A centrally located, highly vascular mass causing extensive septal destruction

44. A nine month old presents with leukokoria. Which finding would favour a diagnosis of persistent hyperplastic primary vitreous (PHPV) rather than retinoblastoma (RB)?
   a. Calcification
   b. Optic nerve enlargement
   c. Retinal detachment
   d. Microphthalmia
   e. Dense vitreous on CT

45. A six year old boy is investigated for refractory complex partial seizures. CT demonstrates a well-defined, hypodense lesion located in the cortex of the temporal lobe. There is underlying bone remodelling but no calcification. On MRI the lesion demonstrates high signal on T2 and predominantly low signal on T1-weighted imaging. There is no surrounding oedema, minimal mass effect and no contrast enhancement. The most likely diagnosis is:
   a. Glioblastoma multiforme
   b. Dysembryoblastic neuroepithelial tumour (DNET)
   c. Primitive neuroectodermal tumour (PNET)
   d. Cavernous haemangiomas
   e. Ependymoma

46. A three year old boy is referred for a Tc-99m pertechnetate scan following recurrent painless gastro-intestinal bleeds. A Meckel's diverticulum is suspected. Which one of the following may give a false negative result?
   a. Recent barium investigation
   b. Intussusception
   c. Urinary tract obstruction
   d. Acute appendicitis
   e. Anterior myelomeningocoele

47. At a routine 20-week obstetric ultrasound scan, polyhydramnios with multiple foci of scattered calcifications are found throughout the fetal abdomen in between bowel loops. Which one of the following is most likely to be the underlying cause?
   a. Mesenteric ischaemia
   b. Meconium peritonitis
   c. Meconium plug syndrome
   d. Necrotising enterocolitis
   e. Gastroschisis

48. A neonate presents with abdominal distension, vomiting and failure to pass meconium. A water-soluble contrast enema is performed and shows a narrow rectum with a cone-shaped transition zone to a dilated, more proximal bowel. Which one of the following is the most likely diagnosis?
   a. Colonic atresia
   b. Hirschsprung's disease
   c. Meconium ileus

d. Cystic fibrosis
e. Functional immaturity of the colon

49. The following constellation of findings in a ten year old girl suggests which of the following diagnoses? Absent radius and ulna, wormian bones within the skull vault, hypoplasia of the distal third of the clavicle and accessory epiphyses of the distal phalanges.
    a. Klippel–Feil syndrome
    b. Cleidocranial dysostosis
    c. Pyknodysostosis
    d. Achondroplasia
    e. Chondrodysplasia punctata

50. A seven year old boy attends A&E following a road traffic accident in which he hit the kerb and came off his bike. He immediately complained of neck pain and was immobilised at the scene. Initial plain radiographs including a swimmer's view fail to demonstrate the entire cervical spine adequately. There remains clinical concern regarding his cervical spine. The next step should be:
    a. Trauma oblique view
    b. Flexion/extension radiographs
    c. MRI C spine
    d. CT C spine
    e. Repeat swimmer's view with traction on arms

51. An 18 month old boy with ongoing irritability and swelling of the wrists and ankles is referred for a series of plain films. Initial images of his wrists show marked metaphyseal cupping of the distal radius and ulnar and increased thickness of the radial growth plate. The most likely diagnosis is:
    a. Rickets
    b. Normal variant
    c. Scurvy
    d. Hypervitaminosis D
    e. Congenital hypothyroidism

52. A four month old infant presents with cyanosis and repeated squatting episodes. Following an echocardiogram, a diagnosis is made. Which of the following is unlikely on a plain radiograph?
    a. Boot-shaped heart
    b. Fullness in the pulmonary artery
    c. Right-sided aortic arch
    d. Pulmonary oligaemia
    e. Enlarged aorta

53. A four year old boy presents with sudden severe right scrotal pain, nausea and vomiting. An ultrasound and colour Doppler examination scan are performed. Which of the following is true regarding a diagnosis of acute testicular torsion?
    a. Normal grey-scale appearances exclude torsion
    b. Scrotal skin thickening indicates an infection
    c. Testicular hyperaemia does not exclude torsion

d. A hydrocoele indicates a different diagnosis

e. Non-twisted spermatic cord excludes testicular torsion

54. A ten year old boy undergoes investigation for recurring morning headaches and visual disturbance. On examination he is noted to be short for his age. CT head shows a complex, partially cystic, strongly calcified inhomogeneous suprasellar mass. On MRI the mass is seen to fill the third ventricle and cause cranial deviation of the fornix. The mass is mostly hyperintense on T1 and markedly hyperintense on T2-weighted imaging. The solid components enhance heterogeneously. What is the most likely diagnosis?

a. Germinoma

b. Pituitary adenoma

c. Supratentorial primitive neuroectodermal tumour (PNET)

d. Craniopharyngioma

e. Chiasmatic glioma

55. A four year old girl presents with nausea, vomiting and ataxia. CT shows a hyperdense mass in the region of the fourth ventricle. On T2-weighted MR imaging the mass is predominantly hypointense and contains areas of both low and high signal intensity. Contrast-enhanced T1-weighted imaging demonstrates a heterogeneously enhancing well-delineated mass that expands the fourth ventricle and causes elevation of the superior medullary velum. There is a moderate amount of surrounding oedema. What is the most likely diagnosis?

a. Medulloblastoma

b. Ependymoma

c. Pilocytic astrocytoma

d. Metastasis

e. Subependymoma

56. A four year old boy presents with a painful subgaleal mass and painful right arm. Radiographs reveal a well-defined ovoid, lytic lesion in the right parietal bone and a further well-defined defect in the left temporal bone. There is also an ill-defined expansile lytic lesion in the shaft of the right humerus. The humeral lesion shows cortical erosion. T1-weighted post-contrast MRI shows that the parietal lesion is associated with an intensely enhancing soft-tissue mass. What is the most likely diagnosis?

a. Leukaemia

b. Langerhans' cell histiocytosis

c. Neuroblastoma metastases

d. Multifocal osteomyelitis

e. Fibrous dysplasia

57. A neonate presents with jaundice, pale stools and hepatomegaly. A Tc-99m DISIDA scan shows good hepatic uptake at 15 minutes, but on delayed imaging at six and 24 hours no activity can be demonstrated within the bowel. Which one of the following is most likely to represent the underlying cause?

a. Congenital biliary atresia

b. Cystic fibrosis

c. Neonatal hepatitis

    d. Spontaneous perforation of the bile ducts

    e. Choledocoele

58. Antenatal ultrasound reveals a fetus with bowel loops seen outside the abdominal cavity and within the amniotic fluid. Which one of the following associated features would support a diagnosis of gastroschisis rather than exomphalos?

    a. Liver herniation through the defect

    b. Fetal ascites

    c. Defect situated to the right of the midline

    d. Defect involving the whole length of the anterior abdominal wall

    e. Associated cardiovascular anomalies

59. A three year old boy is seen in the outpatient department following recurrent urinary tract infections. Which one of the following imaging modalities would be most appropriate to detect the extent of renal scarring?

    a. Tc-99m DTPA scintigraphy

    b. Tc-99m DMSA scintigraphy

    c. MAG-3 renogram

    d. Micturating cystourethrography

    e. I-131 OIH scintigraphy

60. An 18 month old child with anaemia presents with *E. coli* gastroenteritis, heart failure and acute renal failure necessitating dialysis. Blood screen also confirms thrombocytopaenia. Which of the following is the most likely diagnosis?

    a. Pelvic–ureteric junction obstruction

    b. Medullary sponge kidney

    c. Autosomal recessive polycystic disease

    d. Haemolytic-uraemic syndrome

    e. Medullary cystic disease

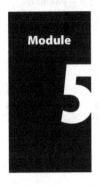

Paediatric – Answers

1. e. Down's syndrome
Anterior vertebral body scalloping is seen in Down's syndrome. Posterior scalloping is seen in syringomyelia, Marfan's, Hurler's, Morquio's, osteogenesis imperfecta and communicating hydrocephalus. In Down's syndrome there is also squaring of the vertebral bodies, and atlanto-axial subluxation occurs in approximately 25% of cases.
(Ref: Dahnert p. 70)

2. a. Alpha angle >60°
Alpha angle should measure >60° in a normal hip. Acetabular angle >30° strongly suggests dysplasia. Beta angle should measure less than 77°. The alpha angle is the line between the straight edge of the ilium and the bony acetabular margin. The beta angle is the angle between the straight lateral edge of the ilium and the fibrocartilagenous acetabulum. Over 58% coverage of the femoral head is considered normal, 33–58% coverage is indeterminate and less than 33% is abnormal.
(Ref: Dahnert p. 67)

3. e. Total anomalous pulmonary venous return (TAPVC)
VSD and PDA will both result in pulmonary plethora and distress, but are left-to-right shunts and acyanotic. Pulmonary stenosis results in pulmonary oligaemia and may or may not be cyanotic depending on the presence of an intracardiac defect with shunt reversal. Tetralogy of Fallot is a congenital cyanotic heart disease with pulmonary oligaemia unless associated with the development of aorto-pulmonary collaterals. Apart from TAPVC, the admixture lesions such as truncus arteriosus, tricuspid atresia, transposition of great vessels, single ventricle and common atrium are some other causes of cyanosis with pulmonary plethora.
(Ref: Dahnert p. 613)

4. b. Centrilobular nodules
The patient had an eosinophilic granuloma and presented with recurrent pneumothoraces due to Langerhans' cell histiocytosis, which is characterised by centrilobular nodules which cavitate, initially forming thick-walled and then thin-walled cysts. The fibrosis that follows typically involves the upper zones. Cystic lesions along the bronchial tree are a feature of cystic bronchiectasis.
(Ref: Schmidt S *et al.* Extraosseous Langerhans cell histiocytosis in children. *Radiographics* 2008; **28**: 707–726)

5. c. Astrocytoma

Astrocytoma of the spinal cord is the most common intramedullary neoplasm in children. They most commonly occur in the thoracic region (thoracic 67%, cervical 49%, conus medullaris 3%). The most common presentation is with pain and sensory deficit but they can also present with motor and gait abnormalities. Plain radiographs may demonstrate scoliosis, bone erosion and widened interpedicular distance.

On MRI, the lesion is usually seen as an eccentric, homogeneous, extensive, ill-defined cord tumour that is iso- or hypointense to the cord on T1 and hyperintense in T2. There is patchy irregular gadolinium enhancement. Tumour cysts and syrinx are also common. Patients with low-grade astrocytomas have a 95% five-year survival.

It is often difficult to differentiate an astrocytoma from ependymoma of the spinal cord on imaging. In this case, the age of the patient, tumour location, tumour irregularity and eccentric position within the medullar favour astrocytoma.
(Ref: Dahnert p. 213)

6. d. Pilocytic astrocytoma

Pilocytic astrocytoma is the most common paediatric glioma and accounts for approximately 85% of all cerebellar astrocytomas in children. Peak age is between birth and nine years old. (Over 80% of haemangioblastomas occur in adulthood.) They are associated with neurofibromatosis type 1 (café-au-lait spots and skeletal abnormalities).

The most common appearance is of a cyst with an intensely enhancing mural nodule (arachnoid cyst should be devoid of an enhancing nodule). They occasionally calcify (calcification is rare in haemangioblastomas).

They run a relatively benign clinical course and almost never recur following surgical excision. There is no malignant transformation to anaplastic form.
(Ref: Dahnert p. 271)

7. d. Multicystic dysplastic kidney

These features are highly suggestive of multicystic dysplastic kidney. The condition is invariably fatal if bilateral, but often asymptomatic if unilateral. It is the second commonest cause of a palpable abdominal mass in the neonate, second only to hydronephrosis. The key features are that no normal renal tissue is present, the cysts do not communicate with each other and they are separated by septae.
(Ref: Dahnert p. 937)

8. c. Lung metastases

Lung metastases are rare in neuroblastoma and are seen in only 10% of cases, whereas they are seen in 85% of metastatic Wilms tumours. Wilms tumours tend to displace rather than encase the vessels, and intrinsic mass effect, rather than displacement of the kidney, is seen. Calcification is seen in 90% of neuroblastomas but only 10% of Wilms tumours. Wilms tumours are the most common abdominal neoplasm in children between one and eight years of age. It typically presents with an asymptomatic abdominal mass but pain, haematuria and fever may be found.
(Ref: Dahnert p. 940, p. 992)

9. d. Ewing's sarcoma

Ninety-five per cent present between 4 and 25 years of age. Sixty per cent occur in the long bones, mainly in the metadiaphysis and have a typical moth-eaten destructive appearance

on plain film. Metastases to the lung, bone and regional lymph nodes are present in 11–30% of cases at the time of diagnosis.
(Ref: Grainger & Allison pp. 1085–1086)

10. **b. Salter Harris II**
This is the most common type of Salter Harris fracture. The Salter Harris classification is a widely accepted and useful classification system for describing epiphyseal plate injuries; these represent between 6 and 30% of all paediatric fractures. The most common site is the distal radius, followed by the phalanges of the hands and feet and the distal tibia.
(Ref: Dahnert p. 84)

11. **d. Lateral epicondyle**
The lateral epicondyle is the last of the above structures around the elbow to ossify. The mean age for ossification of the lateral epicondyle is ten years. The sequential order of ossification starting with the earliest is capitellum, radial head, medial epicondyle, trochlear, olecranon and finally lateral epicondyle. The relevant ages are (in years) two, five, five, nine, nine and ten years respectively.
(Ref: Cheng JC et al. A new look at the sequential development of elbow-ossification centers in children. *J Pediatr Orthop* 1998; **18**: 161–167)

12. **a. Bronchial atresia**
The site and features described are characteristic of bronchial atresia.
(Refs: Dahnert p. 471; Yedururi S et al. Multimodality imaging of tracheobronchial disorders in children. *Radiographics* 2008; **28**: e29)

13. **e. Commonly drains into the left atrium**
Extralobar sequestration is usually seen in early childhood and demonstrates all the above features, but the venous drainage is into the right atrium through systemic veins.
(Ref: Konen E et al. Congenital pulmonary venolobar syndrome: spectrum of helical CT findings with emphasis on computerized reformatting. *Radiographics* 2003; **23**: 1175–1184)

14. **c. Figure-of-three sign**
The above mentioned are plain radiography signs of various congenital heart diseases. The condition described above is coarctation of the aorta. A boot-shaped heart is a feature of tetralogy of Fallot. Snowman sign or figure-of-eight sign is seen in supracardiac TAPVD. Scimitar sign is a feature of partial anomalous pulmonary venous return, and egg-on-a-string sign is noted in TGA.
(Ref: Ferguson EC et al. Classic imaging signs of congenital cardiovascular abnormalities. *Radiographics* 2007; **27**: 1323–1334)

15. **e. Epidermoid cyst**
Both epidermoid and dermoid cysts appear as unenhanced, well-circumscribed, low-density masses. Both can cause scalloping and sclerosis and even destruction of the adjacent bone. Epidermoids do not calcify and do not contain fat (negative Hounsfield units). The presence of calcification and/or fat is characteristic of dermoid cysts.
 Dermoids and epidermoids have low signal on T1 (unless the former contains fat) and high signal on T2, FLAIR and diffusion-weighted imaging. Both may be found in several

locations in the orbit, but most frequently superiorly and temporal. They are congenital cysts but many become evident in the second and third decades.

Teratomas are evident at birth as grossly visible cystic orbital masses. They tend to affect girls, are unilateral and grow rapidly. Conjunctival choristomas (dermolipomas) are less dense than solid dermoids and contain more adipose tissue.
(Ref: Som & Curtin p. 568)

16. c. Fibromatosis colli
This is a rare form of infantile fibromatosis that occurs solely within the sternocleidomastoid muscle. In the vast majority it is associated with birth trauma (e.g. forceps delivery). This is thought to lead to compartment syndrome, pressure necrosis and secondary fibrosis of the muscle. It usually locates to the lower third of the muscle, between the sternal and clavicular heads, and is usually unilateral.

Ultrasound may reveal a well- or ill-defined mass or may just show homogeneous muscle enlargement. In approximately two-thirds of individuals, the abnormality spontaneously regresses by the age of two. Expected ultrasonographic appearances of a haematoma include a heterogeneous mass of mixed cystic and solid components.
(Ref: Dahnert p. 385)

17. a. Choroid plexus papilloma
Eighty-six per cent of choroid plexus papillomas occur below the age of five years and they represent approximately 65% of choroid tumours. Large aggregation of choroid produces CSF at an abnormal rate. This CSF overproduction contributes to hydrocephalus.

The most common location in children is the trigone of the lateral ventricle, the third ventricle is unusual and the fourth ventricle and cerebellopontine angle are more common in adults.

The tumour shows a smooth lobulated border and small calcifications are common. There is intense homogeneous enhancement. Approximately 5% undergo malignant transformation to choroid plexus carcinoma.

Meningiomas are the most common trigonal intraventricular mass in adulthood. They rarely occur under the age of 20.

Cavernous haemangiomas tend to occur in the third to sixth decades and are located in the subcortical cerebrum.
(Ref: Dahnert p. 277)

18. e. Stage IVs
The tumour should be staged as stage IVs. This stage refers specifically to patients less than one year of age with no crossing of the midline and disease confined to the liver, skin and bone marrow without radiographically evident skeletal metastases. It confers a good prognosis. Stage I is tumour confined to the organ of origin, stage II includes regional spread not crossing the midline, stage III is extension across the midline and stage IV includes metastatic disease.
(Ref: Grainger & Allison p. 1648)

19. b. Pelvic–ureteric junction obstruction
Hydronephrosis is a common cause of a palpable abdominal mass in children. The most common cause of hydronephrosis is pelvic–ureteric junction obstruction, followed by posterior urethral valves and ectopic ureterocoele. Pelvic–ureteric junction obstruction is

usually due to a functional abnormality of the ureteric musculature and is found more commonly on the left than the right.
(Ref: Grainger & Allison p. 1541)

20. a. Posterior urethral valve

Posterior urethral valve is a congenital disorder characterised by a thick mucosal fold located in the posterior urethra. It is the most common cause of bilateral urinary tract obstruction in boys. It is most commonly discovered in the neonatal period, but very occasionally may present into adulthood. Diagnosis is usually made with ultrasound and surgical treatment is indicated.
(Ref: Dahnert p. 947)

21. e. Achondroplasia

Achondroplasia does not cause a bone-within-bone appearance. This phenomenon can, however, be seen as a normal variant within the neonatal thoracic and lumbar spine. As well as the above conditions, a bone-within-bone appearance is also seen in thalassaemia, acromegaly, Paget's disease, rickets, scurvy, hypothyroidism, hypoparathyroidism, Gaucher's disease and post-radiation, amongst others.
(Ref: Dahnert p. 187)

22. a. Legg–Calve–Perthes disease

These features suggest Legg–Calve–Perthes disease; this is idiopathic avascular necrosis of the femoral head in children. The peak age group is between four and eight years. The earliest visible signs on plain film include small femoral epiphysis, sclerosis of the epiphysis and widening of the joint space due to thickening of the cartilage. A frog-leg lateral view is useful and may be the only view in which some of the findings are seen.
(Ref: Dahnert p. 51)

23. c. Scapula fracture

A scapula fracture implies a high-energy injury and would be concerning for non-accidental injury. Posterior rib fractures, particularly if of differing ages, are also specific for non-accidental injury. Toddlers who are just beginning to mobilise independently may sustain a spiral fracture of the tibia, sometimes known as a 'toddler's fracture'. Salter Harris fractures are common in children and are most commonly seen at the distal radius and the phalanges of the hands and feet.
(Ref: Carty et al. ch. 8)

24. b. Hypothyroidism

Hypothyroidism causes markedly retarded skeletal maturation – often up to five or more standard deviations below the mean. Other common causes of delayed bone age include hypopituitarism, hypogonadism (Turner's syndrome), Cushing's disease, diabetes mellitus, rickets and malnutrition.

The remainder of the conditions listed cause acceleration of skeletal maturity. McCune–Albright syndrome is characterised by polyostotic fibrous dysplasia and precocious puberty.
(Ref: Chapman & Nakielny 2003 pp. 3–4)

25. **d. Paravertebral**
Extramedullary haemopoiesis can present as uni/bilateral rounded masses in the lower paravertebral region commonly between T8 and T12.
(Ref: Dahnert p. 76)

26. **e. A well-circumscribed heterogeneous mass in the left kidney which enhances to a lesser degree than the kidney**
Neuroblastoma (a) presents earlier and is more likely to metastasise to the liver, whilst this is the right age for Wilms tumour (e) to metastasise to the lung. Haemangioendothelioma (b) presents in early infancy with heart failure. Hepatoblastoma (c) also presents earlier and is less common than Wilms tumour, although it does metastasise to the lung.
(Ref: Dahnert p. 992)

27. **d. Anomalous origin of the right subclavian artery**
The features described are those of congenital lobar emphysema, which may result from all the above apart from anomalous origin of the right subclavian artery, which usually does not result in tracheobronchial indentation.
(Ref: Dahnert p. 478)

28. **a. Right-sided hernia is frequently fatal**
Whilst congenital diaphragmatic hernias are commoner on the left, right-sided ones are frequently fatal. Anterior (Morgagni) hernia is usually smaller and presents in childhood, whilst posterior (Bochdalek) hernia is larger and presents early. Small bowel is the commonest viscera to herniate. Intrauterine diagnosis before 25 weeks is an indicator of poor outcome.
(Ref: Dahnert p. 489)

29. **e. Diffusion-weighted MRI**
The history and MRI findings are suggestive of Canavan disease. This is an autosomal recessive disorder due to deficiency of the enzyme aspartoacylase. Accumulation of N-acetylaspartic acid (NAA) in the brain pursues and leads to leukodystrophy.

   Histology reveals soft and gelatinous white matter. Change is most prominent in the deeper cortex and subcortical white matter, with relative sparing of the deeper white matter and internal capsule.

   On T2-weighted MRI, the globus pallidus is always of high signal intensity, with frequent involvement of the thalamus but with relative sparing of the caudate and putamen.

   The main differential diagnosis on imaging is Alexander disease, a rare disorder which shows no pattern of inheritance. Both conditions are leukodystrophies with macrocrania. Brain biopsy can be used to differentiate.

   Diagnosis of Canavan disease is also possible with proton MR spectroscopy which shows a characteristic increase in the NAA peak. Levels of NAA are also abnormally high in urine and there will be a deficiency of aspartoacyclase in cultured skin fibroblasts. Aspartoacyclase is not present in plasma or blood cells. Diffusion-weighted MRI will add little to the information already obtained with T2-weighted imaging.
(Ref: Atlas pp. 549–553)

30. c. Hypothalamic hamartoma

Hypothalamic hamartoma is not a true tumour by definition. It presents either with precocious puberty or with gelastic seizures (paroxysms of inappropriate emotional outbursts, usually laughing).

The lesion is well defined, arising from the floor of the third ventricle/around the tuber cinereum of the thalamus and extending inferiorly into the suprasellar cistern or interpeduncular cistern. The imaging characteristics described are typical. They do not enhance. (Ref: Grainger & Allison p. 1682)

31. c. More than one episode of vomiting

NICE head injury guidelines for children (under 16) advocate CT head imaging if there are three or more discrete episodes of vomiting. All of the other criteria listed are requisites for acute CT head scanning. CSF otorrhoea implies basal skull fracture. Other criteria include:

- When the head injury occurs as a result of a dangerous mechanism (high-speed road traffic accident either as a pedestrian, cyclist or vehicle occupant, fall from over three metres, high speed injury from a projectile or an object).
- Age > one year; GCS <14 on assessment in the emergency department.
- Age > one year: GCS (paediatric) <15 on assessment in the emergency department.

(Ref: National Institute for Health and Clinical Excellence. *Guidelines for the Management of Head Injury*. September 2007. http://guidance.nice.org.uk/CG56)

32. b. Lipoma

This is a congenital tumour that results from abnormal differentiation of the meninx primitiva – that which eventually differentiates into pia, arachnoid and internal dura mater.

They account for less than 1% of brain tumours but are associated with congenital abnormalities, most commonly dysgenesis of the corpus callosum to some degree. This is particularly likely when the lipoma is located anteriorly rather than posteriorly.

On CT they are well-circumscribed masses with negative Hounsfield units and occasional calcification, and they do not enhance. Characteristically, they are T1 hyperintense and slightly less hyperintense on T2.

Dermoids and teratomas can show similar characteristics, with fat and calcium content. Teratomas may enhance, although dermoids do not. However, the lesion is much more likely to be a lipoma given its position (dermoids tend to be extra-axial (spinal canal); teratomas are much more commonly found around the pineal region, floor of the third ventricle, posterior fossa and spine) and given the association with corpus callosum abnormalities.
(Ref: Dahnert p. 303)

33. a. Prune belly syndrome

Prune belly syndrome is a non-hereditary disorder occurring in males with a triad of abdominal wall muscular hypoplasia, bilateral cryptorchidism and distended non-obstructed ureters. Other associations include malrotation of the gastro-intestinal tract, intestinal atresia, cystic renal dysplasia, vesico–ureteric reflux, pulmonary hypoplasia and cardiac anomalies (including PDA, tetralogy of Fallot and VSD).
(Ref: Dahnert p. 949)

34. **b. Mesoblastic nephroma**
Mesoblastic nephroma is the most likely diagnosis. This is the most common solid renal neoplasm in the neonate. Although definitive diagnosis with CT or ultrasound is difficult, certain features make the diagnosis more likely; it displays infiltrative growth without involvement of the vascular structures or collecting system (differentiating it from Wilms tumour) and only very rarely calcifies (differentiating it from neuroblastoma).
(Refs: Dahnert p. 936; Grainger & Allison p. 1560)

35. **c. Duodenal atresia**
Duodenal atresia typically presents in the first few days of life with bilious vomiting, and is caused by failure of recanalisation of the duodenal lumen in the fetus. It is associated with Down's syndrome, congenital heart disease and other gastro-intestinal disorders such as malrotation, annular pancreas and biliary atresia. The characteristic feature on abdominal X-ray is the double-bubble sign with dilatation of the stomach and duodenal cap.
(Ref: Grainger & Allison p. 1492)

36. **c. Presence of blood flow within the intussusceptum**
The following criteria are associated with a lower rate of successful enema reduction: age less than three months or greater than five years, long duration of symptoms, passage of blood per rectum, significant dehydration, obstruction of the small intestine and visualisation of the dissection sign during enema therapy.
(Ref: Del Pozo G *et al*. Intussusception in children: current concepts in diagnosis and enema reduction. *Radiographics* 1999; **19**: 299–319)

37. **a. Osteochondrosis of the capitellum (Panner's disease)**
The most likely cause is osteochondritis of the capitellum. The blood supply to the capitellum is relatively fragile and osteochondritis usually occurs following a minor injury. The condition usually resolves spontaneously with no long-term complications. Osteochondritis dessicans tends to occur in adolescents and often produces a loose body within the joint causing symptoms of locking.
(Ref: Baumgarten TE *et al*. The arthroscopic classification and treatment of osteochondritis dissecans of the capitellum. *Am J Sports Med* 1998; **26**: 520–523)

38. **b. Idiopathic**
The Scoliosis Research Society has defined scoliosis as a lateral curvature of the spine of greater than 10°. It is idiopathic in 70% of cases. The majority of children who present with idiopathic scoliosis do so in adolescence. There is a strong hereditary component to the idiopathic form. Congenital scoliosis is usually associated with vertebral anomalies such as block vertebrae or butterfly vertebrae. The magnitude of the curve is measured using the 'Cobb' angle, which can be determined on an AP plain film of the spine.
(Ref: Grainger & Allison p. 1593)

39. **c. Enchondroma**
The most common location of these benign lesions is the tubular bones of the wrist and hands, and they are usually asymptomatic and therefore diagnosed incidentally. Of the other lesions mentioned, ABC, simple bone cyst and fibrous dysplasia are rare in the hands. An epidermoid inclusion cyst is most likely to occur at the distal phalanx.
(Ref: Dahnert p. 73)

40. **a. They are often inseparable from the thymus**
Mature teratoma can be seen in the posterior mediastinum and may demonstrate rim enhancement. A fat-fluid level is a specific sign but is uncommon. They may occasionally have a homogenous soft-tissue appearance and be indistinguishable from lymphoma.
(Ref: Dahnert p. 534)

41. **b. Centrilobular emphysema**
All the features described are of cystic fibrosis except centrilobular emphysema. They usually develop paraseptal emphysema.
(Ref: Dahnert p. 492)

42. **c. Presence of three lobes on the left**
The neonate has heterotaxy with right atrial isomerism, which is associated with bilateral trilobed lungs, and both atrial appendages are short and broad-based. It is also usually associated with bilateral SVC and bilateral eparterial bronchus.
(Ref: Dahnert p. 638)

43. **a. A highly vascular nasal mass causing widening of the pterygopalatine fissure**
Juvenile angiofibromas are the most common benign nasopharyngeal tumour. They occur almost exclusively in teenage males. In most cases CT allows accurate diagnosis, although MRI may be used pre-operatively to assess soft-tissue involvement. The tumours typically start in the pterygopalatine fossa and cause local bone erosion. On CT, the presence of a nasal mass and a widened pterygopalatine fissure is pathognomonic of the condition. The tumour may invade the sphenoid sinus, the middle cranial fossa (via the superior orbital fissure), the orbit (via the inferior orbital fissure), the infratemporal fossa, or extend through the sphenopalatine foramen.
  The tumour may be very fibrous but tends to be highly vascular such that it only enhances immediately after bolus injection. Biopsy is therefore contraindicated. Angiography is not required to obtain the diagnosis but may be utilised for pre-operative planning or during therapeutic embolisation.
(Refs: Dahnert p. 387; Grainger & Allison p. 1419; Som & Curtin p. 1579)

44. **d. Microphthalmia**
Primary vitreous normally involutes by the sixth fetal month, but occasionally persists and undergoes hyperplasia. It is the second most common cause of unilateral leukokoria behind retinoblastoma. It may be bilateral as a part of congenital syndromes such as Norrie disease.
  Key imaging findings are micropthalmia (small hypoplastic globe) with an enhancing central soft-tissue band extending from the lens (retrolental) through the vitreous body to the back of the orbit (i.e. following Cloquet's canal). Calcifications are not a feature (cf retinoblastoma – the most common cause of orbital calcifications). Both may show a hyperechoic focus on ultrasound and a dense vitreous on CT.
  PHPV is associated with a small optic nerve whereas retinoblastoma may show optic nerve enlargement due to tumour extension and may also demonstrate macropthalmia.
(Refs: Dahnert p. 350; Grainger & Allison p. 1394)

45. **b. Dysembryoblastic neuroepithelial tumour (DNET)**
DNETs are benign tumours of neuroepithelial origin which arise from the cortical/deep grey matter. They are preferentially located supratentorially (temporal 62%, frontal 31%).

CT demonstrates a hypoattenuating mass and there may be thinning and remodelling of the underlying inner table reflecting the slow growth of the tumour.

On MRI they are hypointense on T1, hyperintense on T2 and small intratumoural cysts may be present to cause a characteristic 'bubbly' appearance. There is minimal mass effect and no associated vasogenic oedema. A third of lesions show calcification and most tumours do not enhance. If present, the enhancement is faint and patchy.

Gangliogliomas and cavernous haemangiomas are other tumours which may cause epilepsy in children. Cavernous haemangiomas are typically dense on CT and commonly calcify. PNETs have a tendency for necrosis, cyst formation and calcification. They also tend to be hyperdense on CT due to high nuclear to cytoplasmic ratio.
(Refs: Dahnert p. 283; Grainger & Allison p. 1279, p. 1684)

46. a. Recent barium investigation
Prior to adolescence a Tc-99m pertechnetate scan has a high pick-up rate for a Meckel's diverticulum. This declines with increasing age as the test relies on the presence of ectopic gastric mucosa, which is less likely to be present in someone asymptomatic throughout childhood. A false negative result is most commonly due to insufficient mass of ectopic gastric mucosa within the Meckel's diverticulum, but may also be seen with barium from recent investigation attenuating the gamma radiation, and dilution of intraluminal activity due to rapid bowel transit.
(Ref: Thurley PD et al. Radiological features of Meckel's diverticulum and its complications. Clin Radiol 2009; **64**: 109–118)

47. b. Meconium peritonitis
These features are typical of meconium peritonitis. This is a chemical peritonitis secondary to bowel perforation in utero. The intraperitoneal meconium characteristically calcifies within 24 hours of perforation. Other features seen on ultrasound include fetal ascites, polyhydramnios and bowel dilatation.
(Ref: Chapman & Nakielny 2003 p. 221; Grainger & Allison p. 1498)

48. b. Hirschsprung's disease
These features are typical of Hirschsprung's disease. This is caused by absence of parasym-pathetic ganglion cells in the bowel wall. Meconium ileus typically shows an empty micro-colon on water-soluble enema and colonic atresia shows a distal microcolon with obstruction at the point of atresia. Functional immaturity of the colon typically shows microcolon distal to the splenic flexure with an abrupt transition to mildly dilated proximal colon.
(Ref: Grainger & Allison p. 1495)

49. b. Cleidocranial dysostosis
Cleidocranial dysostosis is an autosomal dominant condition. Features include multiple Wormian bones, delayed ossification of midline structures, hypoplasia or absence of the lateral portion of the clavicle (10%), elongated metacarpals and short distal phalanges of the hands. Pyknodysostosis is an autosomal recessive condition which also causes clavicular dysplasia.
(Ref: Dahnert p. 60)

50. c. MRI C spine

MRI should be the next investigation in a child of this age group. A ligamentous injury is more likely and therefore CT of the C spine may be falsely reassuring. However, in some centres the availability of MRI may be limited and a CT will often be performed in the first instance. Flexion/extension views should not be done in the acute setting. A trauma oblique view is performed in some institutions instead of a swimmer's view and may be used to clear the cervicothoracic junction in particular.
(Ref: Mirvis & Shanmuganathan ch. 4)

51. a. Rickets

The most common cause of metaphyseal cupping is Rickets. Other features include rachitic rosary seen on chest radiograph, widening and fraying of the metaphyses, coarse trabeculation and bowing of the long bones. The most common sites to be affected are the metaphyses of the long bones which are under stress – ankles, knees and wrists. Cupping of the distal ulnar may be a normal variant but none of the other signs will be present. Scurvy shows a radiolucent band; hypervitaminosis D and hypothyroidism cause a radiodense band.
(Ref: Chapman S. *RITI ELD 5_131 Paediatrics: Abnormal Metaphyses*. London: Royal College of Radiologists, 2009; Dahnert p. 156)

52. b. Fullness in the pulmonary artery

All the above are features of TOF except for fullness of the pulmonary artery, there is usually a prominent concavity in the region of the pulmonary artery.
(Ref: Dahnert p. 584)

53. c. Testicular hyperaemia does not exclude torsion

An enlarged, diffusely hypoechoic avascular testis with an associated twisted cord is diagnostic of testicular torsion. The testicular echogenicity can be normal in the very early phase of torsion. A detorted testis often demonstrates hyperaemia. Scrotal skin oedema and hydrocoele can also be features of torsion.
(Ref: Dahnert p. 974)

54. d. Craniopharyngioma

Craniopharyngiomas (CPs) are the most common sellar/suprasellar region mass in children. They are benign lesions that originate from epithelial remnants (Rathke pouch) of the adenohypophysis and show a bimodal age distribution with peaks at the first and second decades (75%) and in the fifth decade (25%). They are more common in males. If the tumour presses on the pituitary gland, the patient may present with features of diabetes insipidus. Similarly, compression on the hypothalamus may lead to growth disturbance, compression on the optic chiasm may cause bitemporal hemianopia, and compression of ventricular outflow may cause raised intracranial pressure from resulting hydrocephalus. Classically, CPs appear as calcified, mixed cystic and solid tumours with enhancement of the solid component. They may be T1-bright due to proteinaceous components. Long-term survival in children is good (>90%).

Germinomas are typically non-cystic and non-calcified. PNETs frequently show haemorrhage, necrosis and calcification and may resemble the appearance described for CPs. However, they are rarely found in the suprasellar region and are much more common in the

posterior fossa. Chiasmatic gliomas are usually iso/hypointense on T1 and imaging usually defines optic nerve involvement.
(Ref: Grainger & Allison p. 1680)

55. a. Medulloblastoma
Medulloblastomas are highly malignant lesions that account for 30–40% of all posterior fossa tumours. They typically arise from the roof of the fourth ventricle and 75% of cases occur in the first decade of life.

On imaging, they are typically seen as hyperdense midline vermian masses which abut the roof of the fourth ventricle and cause hydrocephalus. There is usually mild to moderate perilesional oedema. Cystic change (high signal on T2), haemorrhage and calcification (low signal on T2) are frequently seen.

They are fast-growing tumours and approximately 20% of cases demonstrate CSF dissemination at the time of diagnosis. For this reason it is important to actively search for evidence of further cranial or spinal disease. Treatment is usually a combination of surgery and radiotherapy.

Subependymomas typically occur in middle-aged or elderly patients. Pilocytic astrocytomas are typically cystic with an enhancing nodule. Metastases are generally multiple and occur in older patients. Ependymomas are usually hypo/isodense on CT.
(Ref: Grainger & Allison p. 1677)

56. b. Langerhans' cell histiocytosis (LCH)
The most common location for LCH is the skull, particularly the diploic space of the parietal bone. Lesions are typically round or ovoid and have a bevelled edge without marginal sclerosis, giving a punched-out appearance. (This is due to greater involvement of the inner table of the skull than the outer.) There may be an associated soft-tissue mass overlying the lytic process which is often palpable.

LCH commonly occurs in children and they present with painful, tender bone lesions. Most bone involvement is monostotic (50–75%) and when occurring in long bones (humerus, femur, tibia), the diaphysis is the primary site.

The differential for multiple lytic lesions in a child include ('FLEM MC'): Fibrous dysplasia; Langerhans' cell histiocytosis/Leukaemia; Enchondromatosis; Metastatic Neuroblastoma; Multifocal osteomyelitis; and Cystic angiomatosis (the last two are rare).
(Ref: Dahnert p. 110)

57. a. Congenital biliary atresia
Congenital biliary atresia is the most likely diagnosis. It has a slight female preponderance and typically presents in the neonatal period. Ultrasound features include a large coarse liver with increased periportal reflectivity. Biliary dilatation is not typical. In severe neonatal hepatitis, the features on Tc-99m DISIDA scan can appear similar to biliary atresia with reduced extraction and excretion. However, the more common picture is one of reduced hepatic uptake.
(Ref: Grainger & Allison p. 1515)

58. c. Defect situated to the right of the midline
Gastroschisis tends to be a small defect (often less than 2.5 cm in length) which occurs to the right of the midline. The herniated bowel does not have a peritoneal lining and floats freely

within the amniotic fluid. Features suggesting exomphalos include the presence of other congenital anomalies, midline defect, fetal ascites, herniation of the liver, amnioperitoneal membrane covering the bowel and the defect covering a large extent of the anterior abdominal wall.
(Ref: Dahnert p. 1044, p. 1051)

59. b. Tc-99m DMSA scintigraphy
DMSA scan is static renal scintigraphy. There is uptake in the proximal convoluted tubules with 50% uptake within two hours and no significant excretion in this time. Excellent images of the cortex can therefore be gained, making it a good investigation for detection of renal scarring. DMSA and MAG-3 provide more functional information.
(Ref: Dahnert p. 1121)

60. d. Haemolytic-uraemic syndrome
Haemolytic-uraemic syndrome is the commonest cause of acute renal failure in children needing dialysis.
(Ref: Dahnert p. 929)

6 Central nervous and head & neck – Questions

1. A 20 year old male presents with the inability to gaze upwards. CT brain shows moderate hydrocephalus and a rounded mass adjacent to the tectal plate. The mass demonstrates marked homogeneous enhancement and is not calcified. MRI confirms a well-circumscribed, relatively homogeneous mass that is isointense to grey matter on T2-weighted imaging. The mass is hyperintense on contrast-enhanced T1-weighted imaging. What is the most likely diagnosis?
   a. Germinoma
   b. Teratoma
   c. Pineoblastoma
   d. Pineocytoma
   e. Benign pineal cyst

2. A 40 year old female is investigated for worsening headaches. CT shows a well-defined hyperdense globular lesion within the trigone of the left lateral ventricle. There is intense contrast enhancement. The most likely diagnosis is:
   a. Choroid cyst
   b. Ependymoma
   c. Colloid cyst
   d. Meningioma
   e. Neurocytoma

3. A 40 year old female presents with bitemporal hemianopia. CT brain shows a large, slightly hyperdense suprasellar lesion. The mass contains several lucent foci and there is bone erosion of the sella floor. There is enhancement post-contrast. T1-weighted MR imaging shows a predominantly isointense mass causing sella expansion and compression of the optic chiasm. The mass contains foci of low and high signal intensity. What is the most likely diagnosis?
   a. Craniopharyngioma
   b. Meningioma
   c. Rathke's cleft cyst
   d. Giant internal carotid aneurysm
   e. Pituitary adenoma

4. When on call you are asked to perform a CT head scan for a 17 year old male who presents with seizures. He is unable to provide a history. A look on the computer system shows that he has had previous regular abdominal ultrasounds and an echocardiogram as a child. Brain CT shows a hypodense, well-demarcated, rounded mass in

127

the region of the foramen of Monro. It is partially calcified and it demonstrates uniform enhancement. What is the most likely diagnosis?

a. Colloid cyst
b. Giant cell astrocytoma
c. Metastasis
d. Lymphoma
e. Haemangioblastoma

5. A 35 year old male presents with ataxia and nystagmus. Blood tests reveal polycythaemia. CT head demonstrates a mass predominantly of CSF density in the posterior fossa. Subsequent MRI shows a largely cystic mass with an enhancing mural nodule. There is surrounding oedema but no calcification. The most likely diagnosis is:

a. Metastasis
b. Pilocytic astrocytoma
c. Haemangioblastoma
d. Choroid cyst
e. Ependymoma

6. A 50 year old woman presents with visual loss. Examination reveals retinal detachment and an ocular lesion. On MRI, the lesion is hyperintense on T1 and hypointense on T2 relative to the vitreous. The lesion enhances post-gadolinium injection. The most likely diagnosis is:

a. Metastases from breast cancer
b. Metastases from lung cancer
c. Choroidal haemangioma
d. Malignant melanoma
e. Vitreous lymphoma

7. A 35 year old previously well female consults an ophthalmologist with a history of progressive loss of visual acuity over several months. Retinal examination reveals papilloedema. Unenhanced CT shows tubular thickening of the optic nerve associated with dense calcifications. Post-contrast injection shows a non-enhancing optic nerve surrounded by a markedly enhancing soft-tissue mass. The remainder of the brain is normal. The most likely diagnosis is:

a. Optic nerve glioma
b. Perioptic meningioma
c. Sarcoidosis
d. Lymphoma
e. Multiple sclerosis

8. Routine first-trimester antenatal ultrasound scan reveals a large posterior fossa cyst and ventriculomegaly. Fetal MRI demonstrates dysgenesis of the corpus callosum, a large posterior fossa and hypoplasia of the cerebellar vermis. What is the most likely diagnosis?

a. Dandy–Walker malformation
b. Dandy–Walker variant
c. Megacisterna magna
d. Arachnoid cyst
e. Porencephaly

9. A 36 year old woman with known polycystic kidney disease presents with a history of sudden onset headache and has signs of meningism. A CT brain reveals subarachnoid haemorrhage with haematoma within the septum pallucidum. What is the most likely site for an intracerebral aneurysm?
   a. Anterior communicating artery
   b. Posterior communicating artery
   c. A2 segment of an anterior cerebral artery
   d. Tip of the basilar artery
   e. Middle cerebral artery

10. A 68 year old male attends the emergency department after being found slumped in his chair at home by a carer. CT head shows an intraparenchymal bleed. On MRI the lesion is hyperintense on T1 and hypointense on T2-weighted imaging. Which of the following stages of haemorrhage best correlates with the MRI findings?
    a. Oxyhaemaglobin
    b. Deoxyhaemoglobin
    c. Intracellular methaemoglobin
    d. Extracellular methaemoglobin
    e. Haemosiderin

11. A middle-aged female presents with unilateral proptosis. CT of the orbits reveals an intraconal mass with involvement of the lateral rectus muscle to its point of tendinous insertion. The lesion enhances post-contrast injection. MRI shows a mass which is hypointense to fat on T2. What is the most likely diagnosis?
    a. Thyroid opthalmopathy
    b. Lymphoma
    c. Cavernous haemangioma
    d. Capillary haemangioma
    e. Pseudotumour

12. Which of the following best represents the decline in positive CT findings for a clinically suspected subarachnoid haemorrhage from scanning at 12 hours post-ictus to 3 days post-ictus?
    a. 90% positive at 12 hours to 70% positive at 3 days
    b. 90% positive at 12 hours to 60% positive at 3 days
    c. 98% positive at 12 hours to 90% positive at 3 days
    d. 98% positive at 12 hours to 75% positive at 3 days
    e. 90% positive at 12 hours to 50% positive at 3 days

13. A 20 year old female is under investigation for periodic halitosis. A CT scan reveals a well-defined, hypodense mass located between the longus colli muscles. There is no enhancement post-contrast injection. MRI demonstrates a midline cystic structure in the posterior roof of the nasopharynx. It shows high signal intensity on both T1 and T2 sequences. The most likely diagnosis is:
    a. Benign polyp
    b. Rathke's pouch cyst
    c. Ranulas
    d. Tornwaldt's cyst
    e. Thyroglossal duct cyst

14. You are called by a paediatrician to perform a cranial ultrasound on a term neonate who requires intensive therapy following delivery. Ultrasound demonstrates a well-defined area of increased parenchymal echogenicity over the periphery of the right parietal lobe. What is the most likely diagnosis?
    a. Germinal matrix haemorrhage
    b. Venous infarction
    c. Middle cerebral artery infarction
    d. Periventricular leukomalacia
    e. Subarachnoid haemorrhage

15. A 14 year old boy presents with a progressive history of gait and speech disturbance. On both T1- and T2-weighted MR imaging, the globus pallidi are markedly hypo-intense except for a small central region of high signal intensity. The findings are more pronounced on T2-weighted imaging. What is the most likely diagnosis?
    a. Leigh's disease
    b. Hallervorden–Spatz syndrome
    c. Wilson disease
    d. Mytochondrial encephalomyelopathy
    e. Parkinson's disease

16. A 45 year old woman undergoes investigation for conductive hearing loss. History reveals several previous ear infections. Direct visualisation with an otoscope shows a mass behind an intact tympanic membrane. Coronal CT imaging demonstrates a soft-tissue mass located between the lateral attic wall and the head of the malleus. There is blunting of the scutum. The mass does not enhance post-contrast. What is the most likely diagnosis?
    a. Chronic otitis media
    b. Cholesterol granuloma
    c. Cholesteatoma
    d. Rhabdomyosarcoma
    e. Squamous cell carcinoma

17. A 52 year old man with known chronic myeloid leukaemia complains of left-sided facial pain. Plain radiographs show a poorly defined lytic lesion centred over the left maxilla. Further imaging with CT and MR demonstrates an enhancing, homogeneous mass with infiltrative margins, which returns intermediate signal on T1 and T2 sequences. The most likely diagnosis is:
    a. Granulocytic sarcoma
    b. Lymphoma
    c. Osteomyelitis
    d. Myeloma
    e. Neuroblastoma

18. A 28 year old woman presents with a mass in her neck. She gives a history of multiple parotid abscesses which have been refractory to drainage and antibiotics. The mass is located at the anteromedial border of her right sternocleidomastoid muscle. Ultrasound demonstrates a compressible mass with internal debris which is devoid of internal flow on Doppler imaging. MRI shows a cystic mass consisting of a curved rim

of tissue pointing medially between the internal and external carotid arteries. There is slight capsular enhancement. What is the most likely diagnosis?

a. Cervical abscess
b. Necrotic neural tumour
c. Submandibular gland cyst
d. Necrotic inflammatory lymphadenopathy
e. Second branchial cleft cyst

19. A 72 year old man from a nursing home presents to the accident and emergency department. Nurses have noticed increasing confusion following a fall six days earlier. His inflammatory markers are normal. A non-contrast CT scan of the head demonstrates a crescent-shaped collection in the left fronto-parietal region. The collection is isodense to CSF and there is no midline shift, nor hydrocephalus. On T1-weighted MR imaging the lesion is isointense to CSF. The most likely diagnosis is:

a. Subdural hygroma
b. Brain atrophy
c. Subdural empyema
d. Chronic subdural haematoma
e. Enlarged subarachnoid space

20. A 40 year old man undergoes investigation for seizures. Head CT with and without contrast shows a large, round, sharply marginated, hypodense mass involving the cortex and subcortical white matter of the left frontal lobe. The mass contains large nodular clumps of calcification. There is surrounding oedema and ill-defined enhancement. MRI demonstrates a heterogeneous mass which is predominantly isointense to grey matter on T1 and hyperintense on T2. There is moderate enhancement. What is the most likely diagnosis?

a. Astrocytoma
b. Ganglioglioma
c. Ependymoma
d. Glioblastoma
e. Oligodendroglioma

21. A 52 year old man presents following collapse. He was previously fit and well, describing only a relatively recent history of dull back pain. Initial CT scan of the head reveals a 1.5 cm hyperdense mass at the corticomedullary junction of the right cerebral hemisphere. The mass shows surrounding oedema which exceeds the volume of the lesion. There is strong lesional enhancement following contrast injection. What is the most likely diagnosis and subsequent management?

a. Glioblastoma multiforme with subsequent MRI of the brain
b. Prostatic cancer metastasis with digital rectal examination and measuring of the prostatic specific antigen
c. Acute haemorrhagic contusion with referral to the neurosurgeons for active monitoring
d. Renal cell metastasis with subsequent CT staging
e. Brain abscess with subsequent intravenous antibiotics

22. Which of the following best describes the appearance of an acute ischaemic infarct of the brain?

   a. Hypointense on diffusion-weighted (DW) MRI and low apparent diffusion coefficient (ADC) values.

   b. Hyperintense on DW MRI and low ADC values

   c. Hypointense on DW MRI and high ADC values

   d. Hyperintense on DW MRI and high ADC values

   e. Isointense on DW MRI and low ADC values

23. A 30 year old female complains of increasing headaches, episodic vomiting and drowsiness. Fundoscopy reveals papilloedema. Non-contrast CT of the head demonstrates hydrocephalus and a globular lesion within the lateral ventricle. There are several small internal foci of calcification. MR shows the mass to be attached to the septum pallucidum. It is isointense to grey matter on T1 and T2. It densely enhances after intravenous gadolinium. What is the most likely diagnosis?

   a. Ependymoma

   b. Subependymoma

   c. Central neurocytoma

   d. Heterotopic grey matter

   e. Meningioma

24. Which is the preferred sequence to use when attempting to identify posterior fossa lesions on MRI in patients with multiple sclerosis?

   a. T1-weighted spin-echo

   b. T2-weighted spin-echo

   c. FLAIR

   d. Gradient-echo

   e. Proton density

25. A 35 year old man attends the accident and emergency department complaining of episodic lower back pain radiating down the legs. History and clinical examination also suggest pelvic sphincter dysfunction. MRI shows a spinal cord mass located at the conus medullaris. The mass is isointense on T1 and hyperintense on T2. It demonstrates contrast enhancement. The most likely diagnosis is:

   a. Astrocytoma

   b. Intradural lipoma

   c. Haemangioblastoma

   d. Myxopapillary ependymoma

   e. Ganglioglioma

26. A 13 year old boy is investigated for chronic headache and visual disturbance. CT shows a well-defined mass in the left middle cranial fossa. It is isodense to CSF. There are no calcifications, no surrounding oedema and no contrast enhancement. There is erosion of the underlying calvarium. You suspect this is an arachnoid cyst but your consultant suggests the possibility of an epidermoid cyst. What MR imaging sequence would best differentiate the two?

   a. Diffusion-weighted MR imaging

   b. Gadolinium-enhanced T1-weighted imaging

   c. Proton density imaging

   d. MR spectroscopy

   e. Perfusion-weighted MR imaging

27. A three year old girl undergoes a CT scan of her head following trauma. No acute pathology is demonstrated but there is basal ganglia calcification. Which of the following can be excluded as a cause of the calcification?
   a. Down's syndrome
   b. Neurofibromatosis
   c. Birth hypoxia
   d. Wilson disease
   e. Congenital rubella

28. The husband of a 33 year old woman takes her to the local accident and emergency department, stating that she is becoming acutely confused and is not her normal self. Her past medical history is unremarkable apart from a flu-type illness a few days earlier. Her GCS is 13 (E – 4, V – 3, M – 6). Initial non-contrast-enhanced CT of the brain shows low-density change within the left temporal lobe. MRI demonstrates abnormal low signal on T1 and high signal on T2 within the left temporal cortex. The insula is involved but there is sparing of the putamen. There is mild mass effect with partial effacement of the lateral ventricles. What is the most likely diagnosis?
   a. Herpes simplex encephalitis
   b. Low-grade glioma
   c. Brain abscess
   d. Post-viral leukoencephalopathy
   e. Dural sinus thrombosis leading to cerebral infarction

29. A 58 year old man presents with impaired vision and intractable headaches. He has a past history of recurrent sinusitis. Examination reveals left-sided proptosis and a palpable mass in the superomedial aspect of the orbit. CT demonstrates a soft-tissue mass causing expansion and erosion of the left frontal sinus. There is peripheral enhancement post-contrast injection. The next radiological step should be:
   a. Referral to an appropriate clinician – you have made a confident diagnosis of a benign aetiology
   b. MRI of the head and neck – you have made a confident diagnosis of a malignant aetiology and wish to stage its local spread
   c. MRI of the head and neck – you are unsure of the nature of the aetiology and want to further characterise it
   d. Perform a staging CT – you are concerned this may be metastatic disease
   e. Perform an ultrasound scan of the orbit – to further characterise the lesion

30. Regarding radionuclide imaging of thyroid cancers, which radiological finding best fits the diagnosis?
   a. Usually concentrates radioiodine – follicular carcinoma
   b. Usually concentrates pertechnetate – papillary carcinoma
   c. Usually concentrates pertechnetate and radioiodine – papillary carcinoma
   d. No radioiodine or pertechnetate uptake but frequently concentrates thallium-201 – medullary carcinoma
   e. No radioiodine or pertechnetate uptake but frequently concentrates thallium-201 – anaplastic carcinoma

31. A patient known to have AIDS presents with increasing malaise and confusion. CT brain shows multiple cerebral hypoattenuating nodular lesions with varying degrees of

surrounding oedema and mass effect. There is lesional enhancement post-contrast administration. Which of the following conditions can be confidently removed from the differential diagnosis?

a. Tuberculosis
b. Pyogenic abscesses
c. Progressive multifocal leukoencephalopathy
d. Lymphoma
e. Toxoplasmosis

32. Which of the following neurological imaging findings would offer a clear differential diagnosis between tuberous sclerosis and neurofibromatosis Type I?

a. Basal ganglia calcification
b. Optic nerve glioma
c. Cerebral astrocytoma
d. Enhancing heterotopic grey matter
e. Multiple foci of hyperintensity on T2-weighted imaging

33. A 65 year old woman is investigated for enophthalmos and headache. She is cachetic, anaemic and you suspect a metastatic process. CT head demonstrates an infiltrative retrobulbar mass. What is the most likely site of primary disease?

a. Breast
b. Lung
c. Renal
d. Melanoma
e. Ovarian

34. A 40 year old man with no previous medical history or medication attends the accident and emergency department. He was the driver of a car that was involved in a car-on-car vehicle collision at approximately 40 mph. He was wearing a seat belt and his airbag deployed appropriately. According to NICE guidelines for head injury, which one of the following criteria alone does not warrant an acute head CT scan?

a. GCS <15 when he was assessed in the emergency department two hours after the accident
b. Haemotympanum
c. Amnesia of events <30 minutes after impact
d. Seizure following the accident
e. More than one episode of vomiting following the accident

35. A 48 year old woman presents with symptoms of hyperparathyroidism. Radionuclide and ultrasound imaging suggest the cause is a solitary parathyroid adenoma. The surgeon requests further localisation with MRI prior to surgery. Which imaging sequence and plane would you choose as the most sensitive for detection of the adenoma?

a. T1-weighted in the axial plane
b. T2-weighted in the coronal plane
c. FLAIR in the coronal plane
d. T2 fat-suppressed in the axial plane
e. Gradient-echo in the axial plane

36. A 30 year old man presents with an orbital frontal headache and visual disturbance. CT head shows a large mass arising from the region of the spheno-occiput and extending into the pontine cistern and towards the hypothalamus. The mass contains amorphous calcification and is seen to cause bone destruction. There is no reactive bone sclerosis. On MRI the mass exhibits mixed heterogeneous signal and a soap-bubble appearance. The solid components show marked contrast enhancement. What is the most likely diagnosis?
    a. Meningioma
    b. Metastasis
    c. Chordoma
    d. Plasmacytoma
    e. Sphenoid sinus cyst

37. A 50 year old woman presents with a palpable lump in her neck. Imaging demonstrates a malignant-looking mass in the thyroid gland. Which of the following findings would direct you towards a confident diagnosis?
    a. Complex mass with areas of necrosis – papillary carcinoma
    b. Calcified lymph nodes – medullary carcinoma
    c. Osteosclerotic bone metastases – follicular carcinoma
    d. Intratumoural calcifications – anaplastic carcinoma
    e. Regional lymphadenopathy – anaplastic carcinoma

38. A 38 year old gentleman presents with a dull ache in his jaw. There is minor swelling over the left mandible. Plain radiographs demonstrate an expansile, multi-locular, radiolucent lesion with internal septations involving the left body of the mandible. It is associated with an impacted tooth. CT shows infiltration of the adjacent soft tissues. There are no discernable foci of calcification. What is the most likely diagnosis?
    a. Odontogenic myxoma
    b. Dentigerous cyst
    c. Odontogenic keratocyst
    d. Ameloblastoma
    e. Periapical cyst

39. A middle-aged gentleman is diagnosed on imaging with suspected laryngeal carcinoma. Which of the following factors would favour a diagnosis of adenoid cystic carcinoma over squamous cell carcinoma?
    a. A history of long-term smoking
    b. Involvement of regional neck lymph nodes
    c. Invasion through laryngeal cartilage
    d. Supraglottic extension
    e. Propensity for nerve invasion

40. Which of the following statements best describes the features of amyloid angiopathy?
    a. Solitary, peripheral haemorrhagic focus in a hypertensive elderly patient
    b. Solitary, central haemorrhagic focus in a normotensive young patient
    c. Multiple, peripheral haemorrhagic foci in a normotensive elderly patient
    d. Multiple, central haemorrhagic foci in a normotensive elderly patient
    e. Multiple, central haemorrhagic foci in a hypertensive young patient

41. A seven year old boy presents with pain in his neck. His mother thinks she can feel a lump. Ultrasound shows a thick-walled cyst with internal echoes. It has a paramedian location within the strap muscles. MRI shows a heterogeneous cystic mass measuring 3 cm in diameter. It demonstrates high signal on T1 and contains areas of low signal on T2. There is marked enhancement of the wall after administration of gadolinium. What is the most likely diagnosis?
    a. Infected thyroglossal duct cyst
    b. Fibroma
    c. Branchial cleft cyst
    d. Teratoma
    e. Lymphangioma

42. A three week old girl is investigated for a right orbital mass. CT shows a diffuse, poorly marginated mass in the superior temporal quadrant of the orbit. It is separate from the globe and the mass shows diffuse enhancement post-contrast injection. On MRI, the mass is hypointense to fat on T1 but hyperintense on T2. On both sequences, low-signal curvilinear foci are seen within it. What is the most likely diagnosis?
    a. Lymphangioma
    b. Rhabdomyosarcoma
    c. Cavernous haemangioma
    d. Retinoblastoma
    e. Capillary haemangioma

43. An eight year old boy with skin hyperpigmentation presents with deteriorating vision and hearing loss. CT shows large symmetric low-density lesions in the parietal-occipital white matter. T2-weighted MR imaging demonstrates confluent symmetric hyperintensity within the parietal-occipital white matter extending across the splenium of the corpus callosum. There is relative sparing of the frontal lobes. Follow-up MRI six months later shows cerebral atrophy and more extensive white matter change with involvement of the frontal lobes and cerebellum. At this point the patient had developed spastic quadriplegia. What is the most likely diagnosis?
    a. Multiple sclerosis
    b. Lymphomatoid granulomatosis
    c. Acute disseminated encephalomyelitis
    d. Adrenoleukodystrophy
    e. Autoimmune vasculitis

44. A 49 year old woman with AIDS presents with increasing headache. T1-weighted MR imaging demonstrates a hypointense lesion in the periventricular white matter of the left parietal lobe. The lesion is hypointense on FLAIR sequencing and is seen to cross the splenium of the corpus callosum. There is peripheral enhancement post-contrast injection. The most likely diagnosis is:
    a. Toxoplasmosis
    b. Progressive multifocal leukoencephalopathy
    c. Primary CNS lymphoma
    d. Cryptococcosis
    e. Tuberculosis

45. A homeless adult male is admitted with a change in mental state and a metabolic abnormality. CT shows a focus of reduced attenuation in the pons. On MRI the focus is hypointense on T1 and hyperintense on T2. There is restricted diffusion on diffusion-weighted imaging and there is no enhancement post-contrast. What is the most likely diagnosis?
   a. Brainstem glioma
   b. Metastasis
   c. Infarction
   d. Tuberculosis
   e. Osmotic myelinolysis

46. A 33 year old male with no significant past medical history presents with headache, drowsiness and confusion. CT shows a hypodense lesion with a smooth regular wall centred over the left lentiform nucleus. There is surrounding oedema and mass effect with effacement of the ipsilateral Sylvian fissure. On T2-weighted MR imaging, the lesion is hyperintense and is surrounded by a hypointense rim and hyperintense oedema. There is peripheral enhancement post-contrast injection, and diffusion-weighted imaging demonstrates restricted diffusion within the lesion. What is the most likely diagnosis?
   a. Glioblastoma multiforme
   b. Pyogenic abscess
   c. Toxoplasmosis
   d. Lymphoma
   e. Metastasis

47. A 15 year old girl presents with suspected optic neuritis. Post-contrast T1-weighted imaging shows enhancement and mild enlargement of the right optic nerve. Several months later the girl re-presents with symptoms of myelitis. Sagittal T2-weighted imaging of the spine demonstrates intramedullary T2 hyperintensity and cord expansion extending from C1 to T1. At the time of the initial and subsequent presentations, brain imaging was normal. What is the most likely diagnosis?
   a. Multiple sclerosis
   b. Sarcoidosis
   c. Devic syndrome
   d. Neurofibromatosis
   e. Ependymoma

48. A five year old boy presents with visual fixation. The ophthalmologist suspects optic nerve hypoplasia. Brain CT confirms optic nerve hypoplasia, an absent septum pellucidum and a third cerebral abnormality. What is the third abnormality likely to be?
   a. Schizencephaly
   b. Cortical dysplasia
   c. Polymicrogyria
   d. Agenesis of the corpus callosum
   e. Type II Chiari malformation

49. A 29 year old woman undergoes a brain CT for severe worsening headache. She is 20 weeks pregnant. No acute pathology is demonstrated. However, an incidental finding of a small right parietal arteriovenous malformation is noted. This is confirmed on

subsequent MRI. You are asked to counsel the patient. What is the most appropriate advice?

a. Normally the risk of haemorrhage is 2–3% per year but this increases by a factor of 10 during pregnancy. Recommend monthly follow-up with brain MRI

b. Normally the risk of haemorrhage is 10% per year but haemorrhage is likely during labour. Recommend angiography with a view to coil embolisation

c. Normally the risk of haemorrhage is 10% per year but there is no significant increase in risk during pregnancy. Recommend annual brain MRI for surveillance

d. Normally the risk of haemorrhage is 2–3% per year but there is no significant increase in risk during pregnancy. Recommend review after delivery to discuss treatment options

e. Normally the risk of haemorrhage is 15% per year but there is no significant increase in risk during pregnancy. Recommend review after delivery to discuss treatment options

50. A 36 year old female presents following a tonic-clonic seizure. Over the preceding months she had suffered with progressive, severe headaches. Contrast-enhanced CT brain shows lateral displacement of the internal capsules by enlarged thalami but no abnormal enhancement. T2-weighted MRI demonstrates a diffuse, contiguous area of hyperintensity involving the thalami, caudate and lentiform nuclei, the splenium of the corpus callosum and the periventricular white matter. There is only minimal mass effect. T1-weighted gadolinium imaging shows no enhancement. What is the most likely diagnosis?

a. Multiple sclerosis
b. Gliomatosis cerebri
c. Viral encephalitis
d. Adrenoleukodystrophy
e. Vasculitis

51. A neurologist requests an MRI scan of a patient with longstanding temporal lobe epilepsy. He suspects mesial temporal sclerosis. What imaging plane would you pay particular attention to and what would you expect to find in this condition?

a. Axial plane demonstrating volume loss and reduced signal intensity of the parahippocampal gyrus on T2-weighted imaging

b. Coronal plane demonstrating volume loss and increased signal intensity of the hippocampus on T1-weighted imaging

c. Coronal plane demonstrating volume loss and increased signal intensity of the parahippocampal gyrus on T2-weighted imaging

d. Axial plane demonstrating volume loss and reduced signal intensity of the hippocampus on T1-weighted imaging

e. Coronal plane demonstrating volume loss and increased signal intensity of the hippocampus on T2-weighted imaging

52. A male patient presents with severe back pain following surgery seven months previously. MRI shows extensive clumping of roots of the cauda equina to the right of the midline, suggesting an intrathecal mass. There is no enhancement post-gadolinium administration. What is the most likely diagnosis?

a. Intrathecal metastases
b. Nerve root sheath tumour
c. Arachnoiditis
d. Extradural haematoma
e. Prolapsed intervertebral disc

53. You are asked to provide an opinion on skull and facial radiographs of an infant. The history provided is recent fall, known dwarfism. The radiographs show brachycephaly, widened sutures, relatively large sella, wormian bones, delayed dentition, decreased pneumatisation of the paranasal sinuses and hypertelorism. No fracture is demonstrated. What is the most likely diagnosis?
    a. Cleidocranial dysostosis
    b. Hypophosphatasia
    c. Hypothyroidism
    d. Achondroplasia
    e. Pyknodysostosis

54. A three year old girl undergoes further investigation for refractory seizures. Contrast-enhanced T1-weighted imaging shows diffuse pial enhancement of variable thickness over the parieto-occipital region of the right cerebral hemisphere. There is atrophy of the underlying cerebrum and the right choroid plexus is enlarged. Several hypointense foci are seen within the gyri and adjacent white matter. There is also bilateral well-defined orbital choroidal enhancement. T2-weighted imaging demonstrates prominent superficial cortical veins. What is the most likely diagnosis?
    a. Klippel–Trenaunay syndrome
    b. Sturge–Weber syndrome
    c. Wyburn–Mason syndrome
    d. Neurofibromatosis
    e. Tuberous sclerosis

55. A 35 year old female presents with worsening headache and facial droop. Her chest radiograph is abnormal. Non-contrast-enhanced CT brain is unremarkable. MRI demonstrates leptomeningeal thickening and enhancement, particularly around the basal cisterns. Enhancement extends along the right seventh cranial nerve and along the optic nerves. There are several small superficial parenchymal enhancing lesions found bordering the basal cisterns. What is the most likely diagnosis?
    a. Sarcoidosis
    b. Tuberculosis meningitis
    c. Carcinomatous meningitis
    d. Lymphoma
    e. Behcet syndrome

56. A 60 year old man presents with back pain and progressive paraparesis. T1-weighted MR imaging shows loss of T9–T10 disc space with hypointense signal involving multiple contiguous vertebral bodies. Skip involvement of T3 and L1 vertebral bodies is evident. T2-weighted imaging shows a large paraspinal and prevertebral mass. An anterior epidural collection is seen compressing the cord. On post-contrast T1-weighted imaging the vertebral bodies show inhomogeneous enhancement and

the paraspinal mass shows peripheral enhancement with central necrosis. What is the most likely cause?

a. Pyogenic infection
b. Lymphoma
c. Sarcoidosis
d. Tuberculosis
e. Metastases

57. A four month old male undergoes investigation for microcephaly and hearing loss. Unenhanced CT brain shows several periventricular subependymal cysts and multiple coarse periventricular and parenchymal white matter calcifications. There is diffuse hypoplasia of the cerebellum. What is the most likely diagnosis?

a. Tuberous sclerosis
b. Sturge–Weber syndrome
c. *Cytomegalovirus* infection
d. Venous sinus thrombosis
e. Congenital rubella

58. A 40 year old unkempt male is admitted with disorientation and ataxia. FLAIR, T2 and diffusion-weighted MR imaging reveal abnormal high signal in both medial thalami, the hypothalamus and peri-aqueductal gray matter. There is atrophy of the right mamillary body. What is the most likely diagnosis?

a. Lymphoma
b. Viral encephalitis
c. Creutzfeldt–Jacob disease
d. Wernicke's encephalopathy
e. Venous thrombosis

59. A 48 year old female presents with tinnitus. CT shows a soft-tissue mass in the region of the hypotympanum. There is irregular bone demineralisation in the region of the carotid canal and jugular foramen, making their margins irregular and partially indistinct. On proton density MR imaging, the mass has mixed hyper- and hypo-intensity signal. The tumour shows strong enhancement after gadolinium administration. What is the most likely diagnosis?

a. Glomus tympanicum tumour
b. Glomus jugulare tumour
c. Carotid body tumour
d. Glomus vagale tumour
e. Cholesteatoma

60. A 62 year old female presents with symptoms of amaurosis fugax. Ultrasound Doppler of her right internal carotid artery reveals a peak-systolic velocity of 2.4 m/s. What is the likely degree of stenosis?

a. 0–24%
b. 25–49%
c. 50–69%
d. >70%
e. >90%

Central nervous and head & neck – Answers

1. a. Germinoma

Germinomas are germ-cell tumours arising from primordial germ cells. They frequently occur in the midline, mostly in the pineal region but also in the suprasellar region.

In men, 80% of pineal masses are germ-cell tumours, in contrast to 50% in women. They tend to occur in children or young adults (10–25 years old). Symptoms depend on the location but the case describes Parinaud syndrome – paralysis of upward gaze due to compression of the mesencephalic tectum. Germinomas may also cause hydrocephalus by compression of the aqueduct of Sylvius, thus patients may present with signs and symptoms of raised intracranial pressure. Germinomas are a known cause of precocious puberty in children under the age of ten years. They are malignant tumours and may show CSF seeding, making cytological diagnosis possible with lumbar puncture. They are, however, very radiosensitive and show excellent survival rates.

Pineal teratomas tend to be heterogeneous masses containing fat and calcifications. Pineoblastoma is a highly malignant tumour which is more common in children and usually has poor tumour margins.

(Refs: Dahnert p. 321; Sutton p. 1748)

2. d. Meningioma

It is rare for meningiomas to occur intraventricularly (2–5% of all meningiomas) but they are the most common trigonal intraventricular mass in adulthood. They tend to occur in 40 year old females.

(Ref: Dahnert p. 306)

3. e. Pituitary adenoma

Pituitary adenomas are divided into microadenomas (<1 cm) and macroadenomas (>1 cm). Macroadenomas may present with endocrine dysfunction but are generally less active than microadenomas. Thus, macroadenomas often present with symptoms of mass effect on the optic chiasm, or if there is lateral extension into the cavernous sinuses patients may present with other local cranial nerve palsies (III, IV, VI).

The differential diagnosis of a suprasellar mass includes ('SATCHMO'): Suprasellar extension of pituitary adenoma/sarcoid; Aneurysm/arachnoid cyst; TB/teratoma (other germ-cell tumours); Craniopharyngioma; Hypothalamic glioma or hamartoma; Meningioma/metastases (especially breast); and Optic/chiasmatic glioma.

In this case, the sellar is widened and the floor is eroded suggesting the mass arises from the pituitary itself. Low-density/low-intensity regions on CT/T1 MRI correspond to necrotic areas and high-signal foci on T1 MRI (found relatively frequently) represent areas of recent haemorrhage.

(Refs: Dahnert p. 323; Sutton p. 1749)

4. b. Giant cell astrocytoma

The main differential for a mass at the foramen of Monro is between a colloid cyst and a subependymal giant cell astrocytoma. The latter is associated with tuberous sclerosis (TS). Renal involvement is also relatively common in TS and patients regularly have surveillance renal ultrasounds. The echocardiogram was performed to assess for cardiomyopathy/rhabdomyoma.

Other central nervous system findings in patients with TS include:

1. Subependymal hamartomas – these are nodular and irregular and can be located anywhere along the ventricular walls but predominantly occur around the foramen of Monro or along the lateral ventricles. In infants, with unmyelinated white matter the lesions are usually hyperintense on T1 and hypointense on T2. The reverse is seen in adults.
2. Subcortical and cortical hamartomas (tubers) – these appear as broad cortical gyri with abnormalities in the adjacent white matter. They frequently calcify but enhancement is extremely rare.
3. Heterotopic grey matter islands in white matter. These may calcify and show contrast enhancement.

Colloid cysts are typically hyperdense on CT and show border enhancement.
(Ref: Dahnert p. 277, p. 331)

5. c. Haemangioblastoma

Haemangioblastoma is the most common primary intra-axial, infratentorial tumour in adults. They are benign autosomal dominant tumours of vascular origin. Approximately 20% occur with von Hippel–Lindau disease. Other associations include phaeochromocytomas, syringomyelia and spinal cord haemangioblastomas. About 20% of tumours cause polycythaemia. Typical CT and MRI appearances are of a largely cystic mass with an enhancing mural nodule. Oedema may be absent or extensive but calcification is rare. Prognosis is 85% post-surgical five-year survival rate.

Infratentorial pilocytic astrocytomas may have very similar appearances to haemangioblastomas but some differences exist that can help differentiate the two. Pilocytic astrocytomas predominantly occur in children and young adults, are generally larger (>5 cm) than haemangioblastomas, may contain calcifications and are not associated with polycythaemia.
(Ref: Dahnert p. 292)

6. d. Malignant melanoma

This is the most common primary intraocular neoplasm in adult Caucasians. The typical age range is 50–70 years old. They are almost always unilateral and located in the choroid, although ciliary body and iris melanomas are not uncommon.

Presentation can be with retinal detachment, vitreous haemorrhage, astigmatism or glaucoma. MRI shows a sharply circumscribed hyperintense lesion on T1, due to the paramagnetic properties of melanin, and hypointense relative to the vitreous body on T2.
(Ref: Dahnert p. 353)

7. b. Perioptic meningioma

These tumours account for less than 2% of all intracranial meningiomas. They occur within the third to fifth decades and are more common in females. They are also associated with neurofibromatosis type 2. They typically present with progressive loss of visual acuity over several months due to optic atrophy.

They are usually tubular in appearance although fusiform and excrescentic thickening of the optic nerve also exist. Tumour enhancement around a non-enhancing optic nerve (tram-track sign) and calcification are highly suggestive of meningioma.
(Ref: Dahnert p. 349)

8. a. Dandy–Walker malformation
Dandy–Walker malformation is characterised by an enlarged posterior fossa (not seen in Dandy–Walker variant) with high-rising tentorium cerebelli, dys/agenesis of the cerebellar vermis (intact in megacisterna magna) and cystic dilatation of the fourth ventricle (normal in arachnoid cyst). Ventriculomegaly is also common.
(Ref: Dahnert p. 280)

9. a. Anterior communicating artery
A clot in the septum pallucidum is virtually diagnostic of an aneurysm of the anterior communicating artery. Aneurysms of the distal anterior cerebral artery are less common.
(Ref: Grainger & Allison p. 1313)

10. c. Intracellular methaemoglobin

Stage	T1	T2
Oxyhaemoglobin hyperacute (few hours)	Isointense	Slightly hyperintense
Deoxyhaemoglobin acute (1–3 days)	Isointense	Hypointense
Intracellular methaemoglobin early subacute (3–7 days)	Hyperintense	Hypointense
Extracellular methaemoglobin late subacute (1–4 weeks)	Hyperintense	Hyperintense
Haemosiderin chronic	Iso/hypointense	Hypointense

(Ref: Bradley WG Jr. MR appearance of hemorrhage in the brain. *Radiology* 1993; **189**: 15–26)

11. e. Pseudotumour
Pseudotumour is the commonest cause of an intra-orbital mass lesion in adults. It is an idiopathic inflammatory condition and about 10% of cases occur in association with autoimmune conditions such as retroperitoneal fibrosis.

It usually presents with unilateral painful opthalmoplegia. It can be acute (more common) or chronic. The former has a more favourable prognosis as it is responsive to steroids. In contrast, the chronic type frequently requires chemotherapy and radiotherapy. On MRI, pseudotumour is hypointense to fat on T2, whereas true tumours are hyperintense.

Grave's disease is the most common cause of uni/bilateral proptosis in adults (~85% bilateral, 15% unilateral). However, involvement of extra-ocular muscles tends to maximally affect the midportion with relative sparing of the tendinous insertions. This gives rise to the so-called 'Coke-bottle' sign.
(Refs: Dahnert p. 346, p. 350; Grainger & Allison p. 1398)

12. d. 98% positive at 12 hours to 75% positive at 3 days
(Ref: Grainger & Allison p. 1311)

13. d. Tornwaldt's cyst
Tornwaldt's cyst is a benign mass typically located in the midline, between the longis colli muscles, in the posterior nasopharynx. They arise as a result of a focal adhesion between the ectoderm and regressing notochord. This causes the creation of a pouch but when the communication with the pouch is lost, a cyst develops.

Tornwaldt's cysts are usually asymptomatic and are picked up as incidental findings. Periodically, the pressure within the cyst increases causing the release of its contents into the nasopharynx. This leads to presentations including halitosis, foul taste in the mouth and persistent nasopharyngeal drainage. Peak age at presentation is 15–30 years.

Imaging features can vary depending on the protein content within the cyst but typical features are of a well-delineated, thin-walled, midline cystic lesion measuring 2–10 mm in diameter. They are hypodense on CT, rarely calcify and do not enhance. They can be high or low on T1 (depending on protein content) but are high on T2-weighted imaging.

Rathke's pouch cysts are located anterior and cephalad to Tornwaldt's cysts.
(Ref: Som & Curtin pp. 1507–1508)

14. c. Middle cerebral artery (MCA) infarction
Vascular occlusive disease is rare in the neonatal period. When present, it is more common in the term infant and usually results from thrombosis rather than embolism. The MCA is most commonly involved. Aetiology includes: traumatic delivery, vasospasm due to meningitis and emboli secondary to congenital heart disease. Ultrasound demonstrates echogenic parenchyma in the distribution of the arterial territory.
(Ref: Woodley H. *RITI ELD 5_093b. Cranial Ultrasonography in Infants: Common Pathologies.* London: Royal College of Radiologists, 2009)

15. b. Hallervorden–Spatz (HS) syndrome
The finding described on MRI is the 'eye-of-the-tiger' sign. This is closely associated with HS. HS is a progressive neurodegenerative metabolic disorder characterised by extrapyramidal and pyramidal signs. The condition (for which the pathophysiology is unclear) results in the accumulation of iron within the globus pallidi and brainstem nuclei. Two clinical entities exist: familial and sporadic. The familial (classic) form shows earlier onset and rapid progression. The sporadic (atypical) form is characterised by a later onset, often in teenage years, with slower progression.

Although the 'eye-of-the-tiger' sign is closely associated with HS, it has been demonstrated in other rare extrapyramidal parkinsonian disorders including cortical-basal ganglionic degeneration, early-onset levodopa-unresponsive parkinsonism and progressive supranuclear palsy.
(Ref: Guillerman RP. The eye-of-the-tiger sign. *Radiology* 2000; **217**: 895–896)

16. c. Cholesteatoma
A cholesteatoma consists of a sac lined with stratified squamous epithelium and filled with keratin – essentially 'skin growing in the wrong place'.

They can be acquired (98%) or congenital (2%). Most acquired cholesteatomas arise in the superior portion of the tympanic membrane (pars flaccida) and extend into Prussak's space where they can cause medial displacement of the head of the malleus and erosion of the bony scutum.

The characteristic imaging feature of a cholesteatoma is bone erosion associated with a non-enhancing soft-tissue mass.

Complications can be intratemporal and intracranial:

Intratemporal: ossicular destruction, facial nerve paralysis, labyrinthine fistula, complete hearing loss, automastoidectomy.

Intracranial: meningitis, sinus thrombosis, abscess, CSF rhinorrhea.

(Refs: Dahnert p. 381; Som & Curtin p. 1184)

17. a. Granulocytic sarcoma

Granulocytic sarcoma is a rare complication of acute and chronic myeloid leukaemia (AML & CML), occurring in approximately 3% of patients. It is a soft-tissue infiltrate of immature myeloid elements. The mean age at presentation is 48 years and most patients present with a solitary lesion. In the head and neck, they have been reported in the skull, face, orbit and paranasal sinuses. Extramedullary lesions have been reported in the tonsils, the oral and nasal cavities and within the lacrimal, thyroid and salivary glands.

They are also referred to as chloromas, a term used to describe their green colour seen on sectioning.

The prognosis of patients with AML does not change in the presence of a chloroma, however, in patients with CML it may represent worsening of the disease as their presence is associated with the acute or blastic phase. Approximately 30% of patients with chloromas have no haematological disease at the time of presentation.

(Ref: Som & Curtin pp. 302–303)

18. e. Second branchial cleft cyst

Failure of involution of branchial clefts can lead to branchial cleft cysts, fistulae and/or sinuses. Second branchial cleft cysts account for 95% of all branchial cleft anomalies. Male and female incidence is equal and the typical age of presentation is 10–40 years.

Second branchial cleft cysts are classified into four types depending on their location. The most common is type II, which occurs along the anterior surface of the sternocleidomastoid muscle, lateral to the carotid space and posterior to the submandibular gland adhering to the great vessels.

On CT/MR the 'beak sign' is pathognomonic. This is a curved rim of tissue pointing medially between the internal and external carotid arteries.

(Ref: Dahnert pp. 376–377)

19. a. Subdural hygroma

This is a traumatic subdural effusion which shows up as a localised CSF-fluid collection within the subdural space. They present in the elderly or in young children usually 6–30 days following trauma. The majority are asymptomatic but patients may present with increasing confusion or headaches. They are devoid of blood products on imaging, unlike chronic subdural haematomas. Subdural haematomas are also more likely to cause effacement of the ventricular system and loss of the normal sulci-gyral pattern.

Normal inflammatory markers and lack of pyrexia lessen the probability of an empyema.

(Ref: Dahnert p. 329)

20. e. Oligodendroglioma

This is an uncommon glioma which usually presents as a large mass at the time of diagnosis. Mean age is 30–50 years and they are more common in men than women. The majority are located in the frontal lobe (~60%), although they can occur anywhere within the central nervous system, including the cerebellum, brainstem, spinal cord, ventricles and optic nerve.

Large nodular clumps of calcifications are present in up to approximately 90% of tumours. Cystic degeneration and haemorrhage are uncommon. Prognosis depends on the grade of the tumour. High-grade tumours show 20% ten-year survival whereas low-grade tumours show 46% ten-year survival.

Although astrocytomas can calcify, the calcifications are rarely large and nodular. Glioblastomas rarely calcify. Gangliogliomas are more common in the temporal lobes and deep cerebral tissues and the majority of them (80%) occur below the age of 30 years. Ependymomas often demonstrate fluid levels due to internal haemorrhage.
(Ref: Dahnert p. 320)

21. d. Renal cell metastasis with subsequent CT staging

Brain metastases account for approximately a third of all intracranial tumours and are the most common intracranial neoplasm. They characteristically occur at the corticomedullary junction of the brain and have surrounding oedema that typically exceeds the tumour volume. Multiple lesions are present in approximately two-thirds of cases and should be searched for with administration of intravenous contrast. Most are hypodense on CT unless haemorrhagic or hypercellular, hence the lesion in this case is haemorrhagic. This lends itself to a differential of primary neoplasms which includes melanoma, renal cell carcinoma, thyroid carcinoma, bronchogenic carcinoma and breast carcinoma. The history of back pain also suggests bone metastases.

Glioblastoma multiforme usually appears as an irregular, heterogeneous, low-density mass. Abscesses typically demonstrate ring enhancement post-contrast and may show loculation and specules of gas. The patient's history describes collapse rather than headache or confusion following a fall, which moves the differential away from traumatic contusion. Although prostate cancer typically metastasises to the vertebrae, it is an uncommon primary site for brain metastases, especially as the lesion described is haemorrhagic.
(Ref: Dahnert p. 309)

22. b. Hyperintense on DW MRI and low ADC values

Diffusion-weighted imaging is dependent on the motion of water molecules and provides information on tissue integrity. It is thought that interruption of cerebral blood flow results in rapid breakdown of energy metabolism and ion exchange pumps. This causes a shift of water from the extracellular compartment into the intracellular compartment, giving cytotoxic odema. This produces the hyperintensity on DW MR images.

ADC values tend to be low within hours of stroke and continue to decline for the next few days. They remain reduced through the first four days and then show pseudonormalisation between four and ten days. After ten days the ADC tends to rise.

Hyperintensity on diffusion-weighted (DW) MRI and low ADC values are not pathognomonic of acute infarction but sensitivities and specificities of 94% and 100% have been reported. Other conditions including haemorrhage, abscesses, lymphoma and Creutzfeldt–Jacob disease have been described.

(Ref: Atlas p. 939; Stadnik TW *et al.* Imaging tutorial: differential diagnosis of bright lesions on diffusion-weighted MR images. *Radiographics* 2003; **23**: e7)

23. c. Central neurocytoma
Central neurocytoma is an intraventricular WHO grade II neuroepithelial tumour with neuronal differentiation. This rare neoplasm tends to occur between the ages of 20–40 years. Patients typically present with symptoms and signs of hydrocephalus.

Imaging typically demonstrates a globular lesion attached to the septum pellucidum. Calcification is considered characteristic, however it may be absent in approximately half the cases. On MRI, the lesions are usually isointense to grey matter and show dense contrast enhancement. It is extremely uncommon to see peritumoural oedema.

Heterotopic grey matter should not enhance, contain calcium, nor be attached to the septum pellucidum. Intraventricular meningiomas are typically located at the trigone. Subependymomas are hyperintense to grey matter on T2 while ependymomas tend to be heterogeneous, childhood lesions that occur in and around the fourth ventricle.
(Refs: Atlas p. 627; Dahnert p. 302)

24. b. T2-weighted spin-echo
Multiple sclerotic plaques can be located anywhere in the central nervous system but typically they form at the junction of the cortex and white matter and periventricularly.

FLAIR is particularly good at locating periventricular lesions as CSF signal is suppressed. In the posterior fossa, however, FLAIR detects fewer lesions than T2-weighted spin-echo.
(Ref: Grainger & Allison p. 1337)

25. d. Myxopapillary ependymoma
This is a variant of ependymoma and is the most common neoplasm of the conus medullaris. It originates from ependymal glia of the filum terminale. Average age at presentation is 35 years and it is more common in men.

T1-weighted imaging shows an isointense or occasionally hyperintense (due to the mucin content) mass. It is hyperintense on T2 and almost always shows enhancement post-contrast.

Intradural lipomas are hyperintense on T1-weighted imaging but they should not enhance. They also tend to occur in younger individuals and usually have an associated, clinically apparent lumbosacral mass.

Haemangioblastoma can also demonstrate high signal on T1 but is also highly vascular, can show signal voids and approximately half of them will have an intratumoural cystic component.

Gangliogliomas are much more common at the cervical and thoracic levels.
(Ref: Dahnert p. 214)

26. a. Diffusion-weighted MR imaging
Epidermoid and arachnoid cysts can look very similar on CT and standard MRI T1- and T2-weighted imaging. Both demonstrate signal intensity similar to CSF. Arachnoid cysts and the majority of epidermoid cysts do not calcify nor enhance. Arachnoid cysts are typically found in the floor of the middle cranial fossa near the tip of the temporal lobe (50%). Although intracranial epidermoid cysts are more commonly found at the cerebellar pontine angle, they may be found in the middle cranial fossa. Both arachnoid

and epidermoid cysts may have associated bone erosion indicating their chronicity. Diffusion-weighted imaging is useful at distinguishing between the two as epidermoids appear bright indicating the marked restriction of water diffusion. Arachnoid cysts appear dark in keeping with signal from CSF.
(Refs: Dahnert p. 269, p. 285; Grainger & Allison p. 1287)

27. d. Wilson disease
Causes of basal ganglia calcification include:
- Physiological aging.
- Infections/inflammatory: TORCH, TB, cysticercosis, measles, chickenpox, pertussis, Coxsackie B virus, AIDS, SLE.
- Toxins: lead, carbon monoxide, birth anoxia/hypoxia, chemotherapy/radiotherapy, nephrotic syndrome.
- Congenital: Cockayne's, Fahr's and Down's syndromes, neurofibromatosis, tuberous sclerosis, methaemaglobinopathy.
- Endocrine: hypothyroidism, hypoparathyroidism, pseudhypoparathyroidism, pseudopseudohypoparathyroidism, hyperparathyroidism.
- Metabolic: Leigh disease, mitochondrial cytopathies.
- Trauma: infarction.

(Ref: Dahnert p. 244)

28. a. Herpes simplex encephalitis (HSE)
There are two main types of herpes simplex virus (HSV) – HSV type I and HSV type II. Type I (oral herpes) tends to affect older infants, children and adults whereas type II (genital herpes) is the usual cause of HSE in neonates.

HSE is a necrotising meningoencephalitis which has a predilection for the limbic system (temporal lobes, insula, cingulated gyri). Characteristically, there are poorly defined areas of low attenuation in one or both temporal lobes/limbic system on unenhanced CT, low signal on T1 (gyral oedema) and high signal on T2. The T2 high signal typically spares the putamen and forms a sharply defined border.

Changes may initially appear unilateral but contralateral disease invariably follows. This sequential bilaterality is characteristic of HSE. Haemorrhage is typically a late finding. Mortality ranges from 30% to 70% but is reduced with early antiviral therapy.
(Refs: Dahnert p. 284; Osborn pp. 694–697)

29. a. Referral to an appropriate clinician – you have made a confident diagnosis of a benign aetiology
This is almost certainly a mucocoele. Mucocoeles represent the end stage of a chronically obstructed sinus. They most commonly affect the frontal sinus (60%), with ethmoid (30%), maxillary (10%) and sphenoid (rare) following respectively. Patients present with symptoms as described in the question.

Increased intrasinus pressure results in expansion and erosion of the sinus walls. There may be a surrounding zone of bone sclerosis. Contrast injection typically reveals rim enhancement, which helps to differentiate from the more solid enhancement pattern of neoplasms.
(Ref: Dahnert p. 391)

30. d. No radioiodine or pertechnetate uptake but frequently concentrates thallium-201 – medullary carcinoma
Types of thyroid carcinoma in order of worsening prognosis are papillary, follicular, medullary and anaplastic.

Papillary tumours usually concentrate radioiodine, follicular tumours concentrate pertechnetate but fail to accumulate radioiodine, and anaplastic tumours show no radioiodine uptake. (Ref: Dahnert p. 401)

31. c. Progressive multifocal leukoencephalopathy
Progressive multifocal leukoencephalopathy affects about 4% of AIDS patients and is caused by reactivation of ubiquitous JC papovavirus. This causes lysis of oligodendrocytes resulting in demyelination. CT shows single or multiple hypoattenuating white matter lesions without oedema/mass effect. There may also be grey matter lesions in the thalamus/basal ganglia from involvement of traversing white matter tracts. The majority of patients show mild cortical atrophy. The condition carries a poor prognosis with death within two to five months.

All the other conditions listed will have various amounts of surrounding oedema/mass effect and enhance post-contrast.

Toxoplasmosis is the most common cerebral mass lesion in AIDS and is two or three times more frequent than lymphoma (the second most common cause of a CNS mass in AIDS). Multiple lesions suggest toxoplasmosis over lymphoma, however when there is a solitary lesion the probability of lymphoma is at least equal to that of toxoplasmosis. (Ref: Dahnert p. 265)

32. d. Enhancing heterotopic grey matter
All of the other features may be found in either condition. Giant cell astrocytomas located in the region of the foramen of Monro in tuberous sclerosis may degenerate into high-grade astrocytomas.

Cortical tubers show as multiple nodules which are hyperintense on T2/FLAIR imaging. CNS hamartomas (occurring in up to 75–90% of NF1) also display these characteristics – they are often termed 'unidentified bright objects'. (Ref: Dahnert p. 244, pp. 315–316, pp. 331–332)

33. a. Breast
Most retrobulbar metastases are extraconal (outside the muscle cone). Neuroblastoma and Ewing's sarcoma are the most common in children and produce smooth extraconal masses related to the posterior lateral wall of the orbit. In adults, an infiltrative retrobulbar mass and enophthalmos is characteristic of scirrhous carcinoma of the breast (invasive ductal carcinoma). Enophthalmia is also considered to be one of the earliest signs of metastatic breast cancer. (Ref: Grainger & Allison p. 1406)

34. c. Amnesia of events <30 minutes after impact
NICE defines head injury as 'any trauma to the head, other than superficial injuries to the face'. All of the other criteria listed are requisites for an acute head CT scan. Haemotympanum implies a basal skull fracture which should be investigated by CT. Amnesia of events >30 minutes before impact would require an acute head CT. Any amnesia or loss of

consciousness since the injury requires a CT scan if the patient is equal to or older than 65 years, has a coagulopathy (including warfarin treatment) or if there is a history of dangerous mechanism of injury, which is listed as:

- Pedestrian or cyclist struck by a motor vehicle.
- Occupant ejected from a motor vehicle.
- Fall from over one metre or five stairs.

(Ref: National Institute for Health and Clinical Excellence. *Guidelines for the Management of Head Injury.* September 2007. http://guidance.nice.org.uk/CG56)

35. d. T2 fat-suppressed in the axial plane
(Ref: Ahuja AT *et al.* Imaging for primary hyperparathyroidism. *Clin Radiol* 2004; **59**: 967–976)

36. c. Chordoma
Chordomas originate from malignant transformation of notochordal cells. They are typically located in the sacrum (50%), clivus (35%) and vertebrae (15%). They may rarely be found in the mandible, maxilla and scapula.

Spheno-occipital chordomas typically affect males and females in equal incidence and the average age ranges from 20 to 40 years. The majority of them demonstrate bone destruction and amorphous calcification. The solid components show variable but often marked contrast enhancement and MRI may show a 'soap-bubble' appearance. Bone sclerosis is rare.

The description given is that of a malignant process. Meningiomas typically affect older females and only rarely (<1%) arise from the clivus. Plasmacytomas tend to occur in an older age group, are more common in the thoracic/lumbar spine and are often osteolytic and grossly expansile lesions. Metastasis is a possibility, although from the description given – particularly the calcification and amount of tumour extension – chordoma remains the most likely diagnosis.
(Refs: Dahnert p. 201; Grainger & Allison p. 1288)

37. b. Calcified lymph nodes – medullary carcinoma
Lymph node calcification accompanied by a thyroid tumour is highly suggestive of medullary carcinoma. This tumour arises from parafollicular C-cells and can cause elevated calcitonin levels. The familial form of medullary carcinoma is associated with MEN II (parathyroid hyperplasia, phaeochromocytoma).

All four carcinomas may demonstrate calcification within the tumour and may also show various amounts of necrosis. Follicular carcinoma typically shows early haematogenous spread and metastases to bone are almost always osteolytic. Although rare, papillary carcinoma can also spread to bone and the lungs. Approximately 75% of anaplastic carcinomas have associated regional lymphadenopathy, however, papillary (40% but almost 90% in children) and medullary (50%) also show regional lymphatic spread.
(Refs: Dahnert p. 400; Grainger & Allison p. 1712)

38. d. Ameloblastoma
Ameloblastoma (adamantinoma of the jaw) is a benign, locally aggressive lesion that occurs mainly in patients between 30 and 50 years of age. They are found in the mandible (75%)

and the maxilla (25%) and are often associated with an impacted/unerupted tooth. When in the mandible, they typically occur in the region of the molars/angle of the mandible.

Typically ameloblastomas are radiolucent lesions that contain septa or locules of variable size, which produce a honeycombed appearance. The margin is usually well defined but when large it can produce jaw expansion with perforation of the cortex. They may infiltrate adjacent soft tissues and show local recurrence following excision.

Ameloblastomas may be unicystic but these tend to occur around the age of 20 years and there is also a very rare malignant variety which can cause lung metastases.

Odontogenic keratocysts, dentigerous cysts, odontogenic myxomas and periapical cysts are invariably unilocular.
(Refs: Dahnert p. 180–181; Grainger & Allison p. 1438)

39. e. Propensity for nerve invasion
Laryngeal adenoid cystic carcinoma accounts for approximately 1% of all malignant laryngeal tumours (cc. laryngeal carcinoma – 98%). Typically, there is an absent history of smoking and regional lymph nodes are hardly ever involved. Eighty per cent of them are subglottic (around the junction with the trachea) but they may spread through the entire larynx. Their characteristic feature is their propensity to invade nerves leading to paralysis.
(Ref: Dahnert p. 376)

40. c. Multiple, peripheral haemorrhagic foci in a normotensive elderly patient
Multiple peripheral haemorrhages (corticomedullary junction) in normotensive elderly patients are suggestive of amyloid angiopathy. Hypertensive haemorrhage tends to occur centrally around the basal ganglia (putamen, external capsule), thalamus and pons.
(Ref: Dahnert p. 233)

41. a. Infected thyroglossal duct cyst
Thyroglossal duct cysts arise from the remnants of the embryonic thyroglossal duct and account for up to 70% of congenital neck masses in children. Typically, children present with a non-tender mass that elevates on swallowing. If infected there may be pain, local tenderness and recent increased growth. Most are midline, although they become more paramedian below the level of the hyoid. Approximately 20% are suprahyoid, 15% occur at the level of the hyoid and 65% are infrahyoid. Generally they are thin-walled cysts and show typical cystic imaging characteristics. If infected or if the cyst has haemorrhaged, high signal may be seen on T1 and low signal may be present on T2-weighted MR images. Haemorrhage and infection may also cause thickening and marked enhancement of the wall.
(Ref: Barkovich p. 556)

42. e. Capillary haemangioma
Capillary haemangiomas are the most common vascular orbital masses in children. They typically present at birth or shortly after. CT shows a diffuse, usually poorly marginated mass which shows diffuse contrast enhancement. On MRI the mass is hypointense to fat on T1, and on T2 it is hyperintense to muscle and fat but hypointense compared to fluid. Curvilinear flow voids representing blood vessels are typical within the mass. They tend to grow rapidly over the first six months of life, stop growing during the second year and then slowly involute over subsequent years.
(Ref: Barkovich p. 549)

151

43. d. Adrenoleukodystrophy (ALD)

ALD is an inherited metabolic disorder characterised by progressive demyelination of cerebral white matter. It is commonly X-linked recessive and boys present between the ages of 3 and 12 years with ataxia, deteriorating vision, hearing loss, altered behaviour and mental deterioration. It is associated with adrenal insufficiency (Addison's disease). Predominantly, there is posterior white matter involvement with the disease advancing toward the frontal lobes and cerebellum. Imaging shows CT hypodensity, MR T1 hypointensity and T2 hyperintensity. Administration of contrast shows enhancement of the lateral margins of the lesions, indicating areas of active demyelination.

Acute disseminated encephalomyelitis is an autoimmune reaction against the patient's white matter. It may present within days or weeks following an exanthematous viral reaction or vaccination. Imaging demonstrates multifocal hypodense (CT)/hyperintense (T2 MRI), usually asymmetrical, white matter abnormalities. Corticosteroids result in dramatic improvement and follow-up scans show no additional lesions.
(Ref: Dahnert p. 263, p. 284)

44. c. Primary CNS lymphoma (PCNSL)

PCNSL is the second most common cause of a CNS mass in patients with AIDS (behind toxoplasmosis). Typical features include periventricular location with subependymal spread and crossing of the corpus callosum. Non-contrast CT may show a hyperdense lesion due to dense cellularity (for this reason it may also be hypointense on T2/FLAIR). There is often a paucity of oedema and frequent ring enhancement due to central necrosis (note this is in contrast with the solid homogeneous enhancement seen with lymphoma in the immuno-competent patient).

Cryptococcosis is the most common cause of fungal infection in AIDS patients. CT is frequently normal and MRI shows low T1 and high T2 signal intensities without enhance-ment in the lenticulostriate region.

Progressive multifocal leukoencephalopathy typically shows bilateral white matter lesions in the periventricular region, centrum semiovale or subcortical white matter, which are hypointense on T1 and hyperintense on T2/FLAIR. There is typically no oedema nor mass effect and no contrast enhancement.
(Refs: Dahnert p. 265; Erdag N *et al.* Primary lymphoma of the central nervous system: typical and atypical CT and MR imaging appearances. *AJR* 2001; **176**: 1319–1326)

45. e. Osmotic myelinolysis

Osmotic myelinolysis is also referred to as central pontine myelinolysis or osmotic demye-lination syndrome. It is classically seen in an alcoholic, hyponatraemic patient in which rapid correction of sodium releases myelinotoxic compounds leading to destruction of myelin sheaths. The pons is the commonest site, although extra-pontine areas such as basal ganglia, cerebellar white matter and thalami may also be involved. Some patients completely recover but the six-month survival rate is only 5–10%.

Brainstem gliomas tend to occur in children and young adults. Typically the brainstem is asymmetrically expanded with displacement/compression of adjacent cisterns. Local vessels may also be displaced. Enhancement is variable.

Pontine/medulla infarcts account for approximately 2% of all brain infarcts. They may show similar appearances to those described in the question but may also demonstrate enhancement. One would expect enhancement with metastasis.

(Refs: Chua GC *et al.* MRI findings in osmotic myelinolysis. *Clin Radiol* 2002; **57**: 800–806; Dahnert p. 273, p. 289)

46. b. Pyogenic abscess
The differential diagnosis for a solitary ring-enhancing lesion of the brain includes ('MAGICAL DR'): Metastasis; Abscess; Glioma/Glioblastoma multiforme; Infarction; Contusion; AIDS (toxoplasmosis); Lymphoma (often AIDS-related); Demyelinating disease; Resolving haematoma/Radiation necrosis.

Classically, abscesses are located at the corticomedullary junction in the frontal and temporal lobes. The most common causative organism is *Streptococcus*. The wall is generally smooth and regular with relative thinning of the medial wall secondary to a poorer blood supply from white matter (neoplastic lesions usually have a thick, nodular, irregular rim).

In this scenario, the enhancing, T2-hypointense rim suggests abscess. Restricted diffusion is also highly suggestive of an abscess.

Lymphoma may be hyperdense on CT due to a high nuclear-to-cytoplasmic ratio and typically shows solid homogeneous enhancement in immunocompetent patients.
(Ref: Dahnert p. 263)

47. c. Devic syndrome (DS)
Devic syndrome (neuromyelitis optica (NMO)) is a severe demyelinating syndrome characterised by optic neuritis and acute myelitis. There is substantial evidence that DS is distinct from multiple sclerosis (MS). DS may spare the brain, the spinal lesions are much larger than in MS and the serum autoantibody NMO-IgG is greater than 90% specific for DS patients and is not detected in classical MS patients.

The proposed diagnostic criteria for Devic syndrome are optic neuritis and acute myelitis plus at least two of three supporting criteria:

1. Contiguous spinal cord MRI lesion extending over greater than or equal to three vertebral segments.
2. Brain MRI not meeting diagnostic criteria for multiple sclerosis.
3. NMO-IgG seropositive status.

(Ref: Wingerchuk DM *et al.* Revised diagnostic criteria for neuromyelitis optica. *Neurology* 2006; **66**: 1485–1489)

48. a. Schizencephaly
The combination of absent septum pellucidum and optic nerve hypoplasia is indicative of septo-optic dysplasia (SOD). Most patients present in infancy with visual disturbance, seizures or endocrine abnormalities (pituitary dysfunction is seen in approximately 50% of cases). Additional abnormalities are often present with schizencephaly being the most common (~50%).
(Ref: Miller SP *et al.* Septo-optic dysplasia plus: a spectrum of malformations of cortical development. *Neurology* 2000; **54**: 1701–1703)

49. d. Normally the risk of haemorrhage is 2–3% per year but there is no significant increase in risk during pregnancy. Recommend review after delivery to discuss treatment options
Arteriovenous malformations (AVMs) are congenital lesions consisting of multiple arteries and veins, connecting as a fistula without an intervening normal capillary bed. The majority

are solitary lesions except when associated with hereditary haemorrhagic telangiectasia. Approximately 90% occur in the supratentorial region (parietal > frontal > temporal).

About half of AVMs present with haemorrhage (intracerebral > subarachnoid > intraventricular), approximately 25% present with focal or generalised seizures and 15% present with headache.

The overall risk of haemorrhage for an unruptured AVM is about 2–3% per year. This increases to 6–17% in the first year following first haemorrhage and then decreases to a baseline level by the third year. Following a second haemorrhage, the annual risk of re-bleed rises to 25% in the following year. An approximate lifetime risk for patients with previously unruptured AVMs can be calculated as 105 minus the patient's age in years.

Current data suggests that pregnancy does not increase the risk of an AVM haemorrhage, however when possible AVMs should be treated before pregnancy. If the lesion is noted during pregnancy and there is no haemorrhage, treatment risks should be considered higher than the risk of haemorrhage, and treatment may be deferred until after pregnancy. (Ref: Brown RD Jr *et al*. The natural history of unruptured intracranial arteriovenous malformations. *J Neurosurg* 1988; **68**: 352–357)

50. b. Gliomatosis cerebri (GC)

GC is a diffusely infiltrative glioma that may be present with or without a dominant mass. It must, however, involve two or more lobes and usually involves contiguous areas. It affects all age groups and can be of varying histological grade. Presentation may be enigmatic as the normal cerebral architecture is usually preserved. Alternatively, patients present with seizures, headache and personality disorders. Prognosis is poor.

MRI findings include diffuse T2 (and proton density) hyperintensity throughout the white matter that usually extends to involve the deep grey nuclei with enlargement of cerebral structures. It is often bilateral and symmetric with minor mass effect and absence of necrosis.

The differential diagnosis of symmetric white matter lesions includes microvascular change, encephalitis, demyelinating disease, vasculitis and leukoencephalopathy. GC is the most likely diagnosis in this scenario as there is involvement of the corpus callosum and the pattern is infiltrative with enlargement of the thalami (cerebral structures). (Ref: del Carpio-O'Donovan R *et al*. Gliomatosis cerebri. *Radiology* 1996; **198**: 831–835)

51. e. Coronal plane demonstrating volume loss and increased signal intensity of the hippocampus on T2-weighted imaging

Mesial temporal sclerosis (hippocampal sclerosis) is the most common lesion associated with temporal lobe epilepsy. Acquisition in the coronal plane is mandatory for its detection. MRI typically shows volume loss and increased signal on T2-weighted imaging. (Ref: Grainger & Allison p. 1352)

52. c. Arachnoiditis

Arachnoiditis is an intrathecal inflammatory reaction which usually results from iatrogenic injury. Previously, it was associated with the injection of contrast agents during myelography. Now, it is most commonly seen following lumbar surgery. Intradural infections (TB, fungal, parasitic) are rare causes.

Radiologically, arachnoiditis appears as nerve root adhesion. Commonly the nerves are clumped together simulating a solid mass, although the nerves may also adhere to the dura, giving the appearance of an 'empty thecal sac'. In severe cases, the thecal sac may become loculated and compartmentalised.

Clumped nerve roots suggest arachnoiditis and the lack of enhancement makes tumours unlikely.

(Ref: Grainger & Allison p. 1385)

53. c. Hypothyroidism
Many of the features listed may be seen in any of the differential conditions provided. However, large sella and hypertelorism favour a diagnosis of hypothyroidism.
(Refs: Dahnert pp. 177–178; Grainger & Allison p. 1707)

54. b. Sturge–Weber syndrome
Sturge–Weber syndrome is a congenital disease characterised by capillary venous angiomas involving the face (port-wine stain, usually ophthalmic division of trigeminal nerve), choroid of the eye and leptomeninges. Clinical manifestations include focal seizures (80% in the first year of life), developmental delay, hemiparesis and homonymous hemianopia. Seizures typically become refractory to medication.

Leptomeningeal angiomas are confined to the pia mater and occur primarily within the parieto-occipital region. There is cortical hemiatrophy beneath the angioma due to local anoxia and usually after the age of two years there is cortical calcification manifesting as low signal intensity on T1 post-contrast images. Other findings include enlargement of the ipsilateral choroid plexus, dilatation of the transparenchymal veins that communicate between the superficial and deep cerebral venous systems, and orbital choroidal haemangiomas.
(Refs: Dahnert p. 326; Grainger & Allison p. 1666)

55. a. Sarcoidosis
Neurologic manifestations of sarcoidosis occur in 5% of patients. In over 80% of established cases, the chest radiograph is abnormal. Sarcoidosis can involve any part of the nervous system, however it has a predilection for the leptomeninges (arachnoid and pia mater). The most common sites for the disease are the basal meninges and the basal midline structures including the hypothalamus, optic chiasm and pituitary. Sarcoidosis also commonly involves the cranial nerves, which may reveal abnormal enhancement on contrast-enhanced T1-weighted imaging. The facial nerve is the most common cranial nerve involved clinically, whereas radiologically, the optic nerves are most commonly abnormal. Dural thickening/dural-based masses may also be present. Parenchymal sarcoidosis can be seen as enhancing granulomas usually located superficially in the brain parenchyma bordering the basal cisterns. Non-enhancing lesions in the periventricular white matter and brainstem are common. Hydrocephalus occurs in approximately 10% of cases.
(Ref: Grainger & Allison p. 1338; Vagal AS *et al.* Radiological manifestations of sarcoidosis. *Clin Dermatol* 2007; **25**: 312–325)

56. d. Tuberculosis
The vertebral column is the most common site of osseous involvement of tuberculosis (TB), usually as the result of haematogenous spread from pulmonary involvement. The lower thoracic and upper lumbar vertebrae are the most frequently affected. It can be difficult to differentiate between pyogenic and TB spondylodiscitis on imaging but several features

favour a diagnosis of TB: multilevel involvement/skip lesions, relative sparing of the disc spaces, large pre/paravertebral collections which are more likely to calcify, subligamentous spread and meningeal involvement.
(Ref: Moore SL & Rafii M. Imaging of musculoskeletal and spinal tuberculosis. *Radiol Clin North Am* 2001; **39**: 329–342)

57. c. *Cytomegalovirus* infection
This is the most common intrauterine infection and the leading cause of brain disease and hearing loss in children. Typical imaging findings include periventricular subependymal cysts representing focal areas of necrosis and glial reaction, periventricular postinflammatory calcifications, scattered calcifications in basal ganglia and brain parenchyma, microcephaly due to disturbance of cell proliferation and hypoplasia of the cerebellum. There may also be lissencephaly, cortical dysplasia, polymicrogyria and schizencephaly due to disturbed neuronal migration.
(Ref: Dahnert p. 279)

58. d. Wernicke's encephalopathy (WE)
WE refers to an acute or subacute syndrome characterised by disorientation, gaze paralysis, ataxia and nystagmus. It invariably occurs in chronic alcoholics but it is caused by thiamine deficiency. Involvement of the medial thalami is characteristic and typically the mamillary bodies, peri-aqueductal grey matter and hypothalamus are also involved. In the acute stages of the disease, haemorrhage, necrosis and oedema are encountered, whereas in the latter stages these regions tend to atrophy, particularly the mamillary bodies.
(Ref: Atlas p. 1213)

59. b. Glomus jugulare tumour
All of the tumours listed in the differential (apart from cholesteatoma) are paragangliomas. They grow slowly and rarely metastasise. Glomus jugulare tumours originate from the adventitia of the jugular vein. CT demonstrates a soft-tissue mass in the region of the jugular bulb/hypotympanum/middle ear space. Local bone destruction is common, particularly of the jugular plate or the lateral portion of the caroticojugular spine. A unique 'salt-and-pepper' pattern of hyper- and hypointensity on T1- and T2-weighted images is also seen. This represents multiple small tumour vessels. They are highly vascular lesions, usually deriving a blood supply from branches of the external carotid artery.
(Ref: Som & Curtin p. 1306)

60. d. >70%
Although variation may exist between different hospitals, a suggested relationship between peak-systolic velocity (m/s) and degree of stenosis (%) is shown below.

Peak-systolic velocity (m/s)	Degree of stenosis (%)
<1.5	0–49
1.5–2.3	50–69
>2.3	>70
None	Occluded

(Ref: Alty & Hoey p. 178)

References

Alty J & Hoey E. *Practical Ultrasound: An Illustrated Guide.* London: Royal Society of Medicine Press, 2006.

Atlas SW. *Magnetic Resonance Imaging of the Brain and Spine.* Edition 3. Philadelphia, PA: Lippincott Williams & Wilkins, 2002.

Barkovich JA. *Paediatric Neuroimaging.* Edition 3. Philadelphia, PA: Lippincott Williams & Wilkins, 2000.

Bates J. *Practical Gynaecological Ultrasound.* Edition 2. Cambridge: Cambridge University Press, 2006.

Brant WE & Helms CA. *Fundamentals of Diagnostic Radiology.* Edition 3. Philadelphia, PA: Lippincott Williams & Wilkins, 2006.

Carty H *et al. Imaging Children.* Edition 2. Edinburgh: Churchill Livingstone, 2004.

Chapman S & Nakielny R. *A Guide to Radiological Procedures.* Edition 4. London: Elsevier Health Sciences, 2001.

Chapman S & Nakielny R. *Aids to Radiological Differential Diagnosis.* Edition 4. London: Saunders, 2003.

Dahnert W. *Radiology Review Manual.* Edition 6. Philadelphia, PA: Lippincott Williams & Wilkins, 2007.

DeCherney AH & Nathan L. *Current Obstetric & Gynecologic Diagnosis & Treatment.* Edition 9. New York, NY: McGraw-Hill Professional, 2002.

Doherty GM & Way LW. *Current Surgical Diagnosis & Treatment.* Edition 12. New York, NY: McGraw-Hill Professional, 2005.

Dondelinger RF. *Imaging and Intervention in Abdominal Trauma.* Secaucus, NJ: Springer-Verlag, 2004.

Grainger R & Allison D. *Diagnostic Radiology. A Textbook of Medical Imaging.* Edition 5. Edinburgh: Churchill Livingstone, 2007.

Haaga JR *et al. CT and MRI of the Whole Body.* Edition 5. St Louis, MO: Mosby Elsevier, 2009.

Helms C. *Fundamentals of Skeletal Radiology.* Edition 3. Philadelphia, PA: Saunders, 2004.

Kessel D & Robertson I. *Interventional Radiology. A Survival Guide.* Edition 2. Philadelphia, PA: Churchill Livingstone, 2005.

Kochman ML. *The Clinician's Guide to Gastrointestinal Oncology.* Thorofare, NJ: SLACK Incorporated, 2005.

Lee JKT *et al. Computed Body Tomography with MRI Correlation.* Edition 4. Philadelphia, PA: Lippincott Williams & Wilkins, 2005.

Mirvis SE & Shanmuganathan K. *Imaging in Trauma and Critical Care.* Edition 2. Philadelphia, PA: Saunders, 2003.

Moore KL. *Clinically Oriented Anatomy.* Edition 3. Philadelphia, PA: Lippincott Williams & Wilkins, 1992.

Osborn AG. *Diagnostic Neuroradiology.* St Louis, MO: Mosby, 1993.

Rogers L. *Radiology of Skeletal Trauma.* Edition 3. Philadelphia, PA: Churchill Livingstone, 2001.

Saclarides TJ *et al. Surgical Oncology: An Algorithmic Approach.* New York, NY: Springer, 2003.

Silverman SG & Cohan RH. *CT Urography: An Atlas.* Philadelphia, PA: Lippincott Williams & Wilkins, 2006.

Som PM & Curtin HD. *Head and Neck Imaging.* Edition 4. St Louis, MO: Mosby, 2003.

Stevenson RE & Hall JG. *Human Malformations and Related Anomalies.* Edition 2. New York, NY: Oxford University Press, 2006.

Sutton D. *Textbook of Radiology and Imaging.* Edition 7. Edinburgh: Churchill Livingstone, 2003.

Weissleder R *et al. Primer of Diagnostic Imaging.* Edition 4. St Louis, MO: Mosby, 2006.

Zagoria RJ. *Genitourinary Radiology: The Requisites.* Edition 2. Philadelphia, PA: Elsevier Health Sciences, 2004.

Index

Printed in the United States
by Baker & Taylor Publisher Services